CONTROVERSIES IN NEUROLOGY

Controversies in Neurology

Editors

Richard A. Thompson, M.D.
Division of Neurology
Barrow Neurological Institute
St. Joseph's Hospital and Medical Center
Phoenix, Arizona

John R. Green, M.D., FACS
Chairman, Barrow Neurological Institute
St. Joseph's Hospital and Medical Center
Phoenix, Arizona

Raven Press ■ New York

Preface

This volume brings together specialists in areas of neurology and neurosurgery where there are presently no clearcut guidelines for management. In their discussions of controversial subjects that require further evaluation, such as the place of manipulation therapy in the conservative management of cervical problems, emphasis is placed upon recent developments in the field in question and an attempt is made to reach a consensus on the optimal approach to treatment.

Topics discussed include the surgical approach to the management of spondylosis and stenosis, the management of cervical disc disease with and without fusion, and the problems of managing stenosis of the carotid arteries with anticoagulant and antiplatelet treatment. Metastatic spinal cord tumors and tumors of the brain are discussed in considerable detail, and a variety of interesting cases are presented. Concluding with guidelines for the management and treatment of arteriovenous malformations and aneurysms, this volume will be of interest to all neurologists, neurosurgeons and orthopedic surgeons.

R.H. Thompson, M.D.
J.R. Green, M.D.

Acknowledgments

We are indebted to the internationally recognized authors who have contributed to this volume and to the excellent symposium on which it is based.

Richard A. Thompson, M.D., Chairman

Robert M. Crowell, M.D.

John R. Green, M.D., FACS

William B. Helme, M.D.

John A. Hodak, M.D.

Daniel A. Pollen, M.D.

John D. Waggener, M.D.

Joseph C. White, M.D.

Elizabeth Wilkinson, M.D.

The Symposium Committee

Contents

Contributors

William W. Anderson
Neurological Medical Group
Burlingame, California 94010

H. J. M. Barnett
University Hospital
University of Western Ontario
London, Ontario, Canada N6A 5A5

Robert M. Crowell
Barrow Neurological Institute
St. Joseph's Hospital and Medical Center
Phoenix, Arizona 85013

John J. Demakas
Barrow Neurological Institute
St. Joseph's Hospital and Medical Center
Phoenix, Arizona 85013

John R. Green
Barrow Neurological Institute
St. Joseph's Hospital and Medical Center
Phoenix, Arizona 85013

Philip H. Gutin
Brain Tumor Research Center and the
    Departments of Neurological Surgery
    and Radiation Oncology
School of Medicine
University of California, San Francisco
San Francisco, California 94143

J. Philip Kistler
Neurology Service
Massachusetts General Hospital
Harvard Medical School
Boston, Massachusetts 02114

Victor A. Levin
Brain Tumor Research Center and the
    Departments of Neurological Surgery
    and Radiation Oncology
School of Medicine
University of California, San Francisco
San Francisco, California 94143

Sean Mullan
University of Chicago Hospitals
Chicago, Illinois 60637

Robert J. Ojemann
Neurology Service
Massachusetts General Hospital
Harvard Medical School
Boston, Massachusetts 02114

Russel H. Patterson, Jr.
525 East 68th Street
New York, New York 10021

Apichan Pootrakul
Barrow Neurological Institute
St. Joseph's Hospital and Medical Center
Phoenix, Arizona 85013

Jerome B. Posner
Department of Neurology
Memorial Sloan-Kettering Cancer Center
New York, New York 10021

James T. Robertson
Department of Neurosurgery
The University of Tennessee Center for
    the Health Sciences
Memphis, Tennessee 38163

William R. Shapiro
Department of Neurology
Memorial Sloan-Kettering Cancer Center
New York, New York 10021

John M. Tew, Jr.
Mayfield Neurological Institute
Cincinnati, Ohio 45220

Philip R. Weinstein
Section of Neurosurgery
Arizona Health Sciences Center
Tucson, Arizona 85724

Controversies in Neurology, edited by R. A.
Thompson and J. R. Green. Raven Press,
New York © 1983.

Cervical Spine Disease: Conservative Management and Manipulation Therapy

William W. Anderson

Neurological Medical Group, Burlingame, California 94010

The use of manipulation in the treatment of cervical discs has received little attention from the medical profession. This form of therapy has not been ignored by the public who seek this form of treatment from nonmedical practitioners with increasing frequency. There is a small group of physicians in the United States who use such techniques, however they generally are ignored or ridiculed by their colleagues. On the other hand, many physicians, including myself, have been less than happy with the results of the present treatment for patients with so-called whiplash injuries, cervicoscapular pain, or chronic cervical pain. The present treatment is prolonged and expensive, and the results in a large number of cases are less than optimal. After a few weeks of medical treatment, many patients seek out a lay practitioner, usually a chiropractor, for a more definitive treatment which almost invariably includes manipulation.

There are four different schools of thought concerning the use of manipulation to treat musculoskeletal disorders.

1. *Osteopathy.* Today, most osteopathic physicians in the U.S. receive training not unlike that received in U.S. medical schools. Osteopathic students are no longer taught that all maladies are due to disease of the spine and its nerves, as was claimed in the past. Osteopathic treatment for musculoskeletal disorders is based on the theory that there is reduced spinal mobility. Treatment attempts to restore a full range of motion to the spinal joint (1,4,5).

2. *Chiropractic theory.* The basis of chiropractic treatment is the theory that all disease, including musculoskeletal problems, is due to malalignment of vertebral bodies. Their treatment attempts to shift the vertebrae back into place. Physicians have deplored these practices for decades, and rightly so. Needless to say, chiropractors have been very successful in convincing the federal government, industrial insurance companies, and the legislatures of all 50 states of the merits of their particular health care delivery system. By ignoring the use of manipulation, the medical profession has, by default, left its use to nonmedical practitioners, particularly to the chiropractic profession.

3. *Oscillatory techniques.* Originally described about 160 years ago, oscillatory techniques now have a wide following among physiotherapists in this country. Their

foremost advocate is Maitland. The method of treatment uses small, repetitive movements of the involved joint to restore complete mobility.

4. *Neuro-orthopedic methods.* The neuro-orthopedic methods of Dr. James Cyriax[1] (2,3) are based on the theory that most pain in the cervical area is due to displacement of a fragment of a disc. Under certain conditions, the disc fragment may be manipulated back into place. All manipulations are carried out under strong manual traction with an assistant holding the patient's legs, after a complete neurological examination as well as a complete examination of the mobility of the cervical spine. I shall confine myself in this chapter to Dr. Cyriax's methods, since I believe his techniques of evaluating patients, and the criteria he uses in deciding for or against manipulation, have much merit.

In addition to a complete neurological examination, a careful evaluation of the mobility of the cervical and thoracic spine is carried out. The reason the thoracic spine and shoulders are examined is that upper thoracic pain can be referred to the cervical spine and vice versa. Likewise, pain originating from the shoulder, such as an acute bursitis, can radiate down an arm as far as the wrist and up as far as the side of the neck. If the origin of the pain is the shoulder, treatment should be directed there. Manipulation of the cervical spine in that situation is useless.

The examination recommended by Dr. Cyriax includes active and passive range of movement as well as resistive movements in the evaluation of the musculoskeletal system. The same evaluation is carried out whether the pain is in the lumbar, thoracic, or cervical area.

RANGE OF MOTION

Normally, the range of motion of the cervical vertebrae is as follows: (a) flexion and extension—80°, (b) lateral rotation—80 to 90°, (c) side flexion—60°.

Naturally, in elderly people, there may be considerable limitation in the range of motion whether they are symptomatic or not.

Active Range of Motion of the Neck

The patient is asked to turn his head as far as he can in the following six planes:
a) head right
b) head left
c) side flexion right
d) side flexion left
e) head back
f) head forward

The physician asks the patient which, if any, of these maneuvers alters the pain in any way. The patient's responses are duly recorded.

---

[1] Formerly Head, Department of Physiotherapy, Saint Thomas Hospital Medical School, London.

Passive Range of Motion of the Neck

Passive range of motion of the neck is then tested and is carried out in the same six planes. The patient relaxes his neck muscles while the range of movement of the neck is ascertained by the physician gently moving the neck in the same six planes. The active and passive range of movements should be the same. The examiner must note the type of resistance he feels at the extreme range of motion. This is what is called the "end feel." The common types of end feel noted during passive movements are as follows:

a) Bone-to-bone, such as one normally notes on extreme passive extension of the elbow. If the end feel is bone-to-bone, manipulation is useless.

b) The capsular feel, which is not unlike a piece of leather being stretched. It is this type of end feel that must be present if manipulation is to work.

c) Muscle spasm, when suddenly it is noted that severe muscle spasm occurs and the neck will not move. If this is present, manipulation is contraindicated as it will not work since the pain is of muscular rather than bone-cartilage origin.

d) The empty feel, in which the patient has severe pain long before normal range of motion is obtained. There is no bone-to-bone resistance, yet the patient is obviously in severe pain. Usually this type of end feel indicates metastatic neoplasm or possibly a localized infectious process in the cervical vertebrae. Manipulation is therefore contraindicated.

Resisted Range of Motion

The patient is asked to push his head against the physician's hand in the same six planes. The physician applies counter pressure so that no movement occurs. If the patient's problem is muscular in origin, one or more of the resistive movements will increase his pain. If the origin of the pain is in the cervical spine, there should be no increase in pain since the vertebrae should be immobile during this part of the examination.

Commonly in pain due to a cervical disc derangement, the following phenomena will be noted: The pain will be increased during the active and passive movements of the neck in two, three, or four movements of the six neck maneuvers, and will be unaffected by four, three, or two movements. Active rotation to the side of the pain will invariably hurt. Usually, one or both side flexions will also hurt. The pain is increased by the same two, three, or four movements in both the active and passive maneuvers in cervical disc lesions. The pain is somewhat more severe on passive range of motion; likewise, the range of motion is slightly more than the active movements. The resisted movements should not alter the pain since there is no movement of the cervical vertebrae. If active, passive, and resistive movements all hurt, the patient's problem is usually non-organic.

Examination of the thoracic spine consists of the following maneuvers. The patient stands with his back facing the examiner. The physician notes any changes in the normal anatomy of the thoracic and lumbar spine. The patient is then tested for the following active, passive, and resistive movements:

a) adduction of the scapula, which will tend to pull on nerve roots T1 and T2,
b) abduction of the scapula,
c) elevation of the shoulders,
d) left lateral side flexion,
e) right lateral side flexion,
f) flexion of the thoracic spine,
g) extension of the thoracic spine,
h) right lateral rotation, and
i) left lateral rotation.

Shoulder examination is carried out in the active, passive, and resistive range in the following maneuvers:

a) elevation of the shoulder,
b) scapulohumeral range of abduction (normal range is 85° to 110°),
c) lateral rotation of the shoulder,
d) medial rotation of the shoulder,
e) flexion of the forearm, and
f) extension of the forearm.

If only the thoracic and/or shoulder maneuvers reproduce or aggravate the pain, then the patient is not a candidate for manual traction. If the neck signs are normal and the shoulder signs are positive, then the origin of the pain is in the shoulder and referred to the neck. Since the neck is immobile during the shoulder and thoracic maneuvers, any reproduction or enhancement of the pain must be coming from the shoulder since this is the only part that is moving.

INDICATIONS AND CONTRAINDICATIONS FOR MANIPULATION OF THE CERVICAL SPINE

After a complete neurological examination and assessment of the results of the standard neurological examination, as well as the examination of the musculoskeletal system, the physician determines which bony part is the origin of the pain. If it appears to be the cervical spine and an articular pattern is present, the patient may be a candidate for manipulation.

Contraindications for manipulation are (a) evidence of any long-tract signs, (b) a history suggestive of basilar artery insufficiency, (c) anticoagulant use, (d) significant weakness of a muscle or group of muscles in the upper limbs, (d) the absence of articular signs on the six active and passive movements of the neck, (f) evidence of gross deformity of the cervical vertebrae on X-ray, (g) increased pain down the arm or the production of long-tract signs during an attempt at manual traction (which is then discontinued), (h) spasmodic torticollis, and (i) rheumatoid arthritis of the cervical vertebrae.

Indications for manipulation are the absence of the contraindications and the presence of a partial articular pattern.

In brief, patients with the following symptoms (and in whom a partial articular pattern is present) do well with manipulation: pain in the back of the neck, radiating to the scapula and/or shoulder without any arm or forearm pain; unilateral scapular and root pain above the elbow; and absence of increasing pain with neck movements.

Patients with the symptoms below may or may not benefit from manual traction: unilateral scapular and root pain with increasing pain with neck movements; bilateral scapular and arm pain with minimal evidence of an articular pattern during active and resistive range of motion of the neck; questionable evidence of muscle weakness; and brachial pain that begins in the forearm with paresthetic fingers.

Manipulation is never carried out under anesthesia because one can never assess how much relief of pain the patient has had after each manipulation. If the patient were to develop neurological signs, one would be unaware of this during general anesthesia. Manipulation is a painless procedure.

All cervical manipulations are carried out under traction with the physician using his full body weight. X-ray evidence has shown that between each cervical vertebra, there is an additional 2.5 mm of space between the discs when a force between 100 to 140 kg is applied by the examiner.

It is felt that manual traction works for the following reasons:

a) The pressure in the displaced cartilaginous portion of the disc eases, and therefore the pain abates.

b) The vertebra interspaces are enlarged.

c) The facet joints are disengaged and, thus, more movement is possible at the intervertebral joint.

d) The suction effect of manual traction may help to cause the disc fragment to move back into place.

While the patient lies on a flat table elevated 36 inces, straight manual traction with the neck in slight extension is carried out. The physician has an attendant hold the patient's feet and uses his body weight as leverage until he feels the neck muscles relax. Once this has occurred, the appropriate movement is carried out until a small click is heard. The patient is then asked to sit up and to move his neck in the same six directions, while the range of motion and the amount of pain the patient is experiencing after manipulation are assessed. The standard manipulations for patients who meet the criteria are:

a) Straight horizontal traction. As the neck muscles relax, slow rotatory movements from side to side are carried out. This maneuver is repeated as long as it seems to give some relief of pain.

b) Traction with less than full range to the side which does not hurt. This maneuver is repeated as long as the pain recedes. When it stops improving, then one goes on to the next maneuver.

c) Rotation to full range to the painless side.

(d) Rotation three-quarters of the way to the side that hurts.

e) Full rotation to the side that hurts.

f) Side flexion toward the painless side.

g) Lateral or anterior-posterior (A–P) glide with gradual rocking of the head from side to side or flexion and extension.

It has been my experience that the straight A–P pull as well as rotation to the side of the pain will usually relieve the pain in 40% of cases. Remember, it is important to repeat any maneuver that decreases the patient's pain until it seems the improvement has stabilized. The physician must have the patient go through the six neck movements after every manipulation so that he can assess the range of movement of the neck and any change in the pain pattern. If the physician finds that one maneuver aggravates the pain, then he shouldn't repeat that maneuver but go ont to the next one.

SUMMARY

In summary, many patients with neck and arm pain but without neurological findings can be readily cured by manipulation. One should carefully select one's cases and be able to carry out a complete neurological and musculoskeletal examination to be certain the pain is coming from the cervical spine and not from the upper thoracic spine and/or shoulder.

Even should manipulation be decided against, Dr. Cyriax's methods of examining the musculoskeletal system are valuable for their improvement of diagnostic acumen and their precision in localizing the site of the pain. It also is an almost foolproof method of separating the neurotic patient from the one who has genuine organic disease without significant neurological findings.

REFERENCES

1. Edwards, B. C. (1979): Australian association of manipulative medicine. *Med. J. Aust.*, 1:116–117.
2. Cyriax, J., and Gillian, W. (1977): *Textbook of Orthopaedic Medicine*, Vol. 2, 9th ed., William & Wilkins Co., Baltimore.
3. Cyriax, J. (1978): *Textbook of Orthopaedic Medicine*, Vol. I, 7th ed., Williams & Wilkins Co., Baltimore.
4. Gorman, R. F. (1978): Cardiac arrest after cervical spine mobilization. *Med. J. Aust.*, 2:169–170.
5. Winer, C. D. (1979): Spinal manipulation for migraine. *Aust. J. Med.*, 9:340–342.

Surgical Approach to Cervical Spondylosis and Stenosis

Philip R. Weinstein

Section of Neurosurgery, Arizona Health Sciences Center, Tucson, Arizona 85724

Although radiculomyelopathy due to cervical spondylosis is the most common spinal cord disease after the age of 40, there are as yet many controversies as to when and why decompressive surgery is indicated and how it should best be performed (6). The pathogenesis of cervical spinal stenosis remains unexplained, and the mechanisms of spinal cord and nerve root dysfunction are multiple. Correlation is often poor between radiographic findings and the extent or level of neurological deficit. The differential diagnosis includes degenerative as well as neoplastic disorders. The role of minor trauma is poorly understood, and vulnerability to future problems at other spinal levels is unpredictable. Surgeons must choose and tailor the appropriate anterior or posterior or lateral approach for decompression with or without fusion. Results of surgical treatment are difficult to predict in the individual case, especially with advanced cases of quadriparesis or amyotrophy. Therefore, review of these controversial issues, in the light of recent clinical experience and laboratory research, is of considerable interest to clinicians dealing with cervical spine disorders.

PATHOGENESIS

Stenosis

The dimensions and shape of the cervical spinal canal are known to vary significantly on a developmental basis (3,23,37,56). The sagittal canal diameter may be 70% larger in spines at the upper end of the range of individual variation (11,57). The mean diameter at the C_3 to C_7 levels measured from the center of concavity of the posterior surface of the vertebral bodies to the point of dorsal junction of the two lamina with the spinous process (spinolaminar line) is 17 ± 5 mm (11). Measuring from the vertebral body marginal osteophyte usually reveals the smallest sagittal diameter (Fig. 4A). When the sagittal cervical canal diameter is 10 mm or less, neurological deficit due to compressive myelopathy is inevitable (6). With diameters of 10 to 12 mm, symptomatic entrapment of the cord is probable, but when the bony canal measures 13 mm or more, cord dysfunction due to spinal stenosis is unlikely (71). Measurements show little difference within individual spines from C_4 to C_7, although normal average values at C_1 are 22 to 23 mm, and at C_2 to C_3 they are 18 to 20 mm (45,79). Sagittal diameters of less then 14 mm are rare, falling below two standard deviations at a given cervical segment (42,45). In two radiological surveys of series of 300 and 200 normal subjects, incidence rates for such cervical stenosis of 0.3% and 1% were found (11,79).

However, although developmental stenosis of the cervical spinal canal is rare, it is a predisposing factor in patients with symptomatic cervical spondylosis (27,52,76). In fact, cervical spondylosis alone is usually a neurologically asymptomatic condition observed incidentally on radiographs in over 50% of individuals over the age of 50 (10,25). Hypertrophic degenerative joint alterations and osteophyte proliferation, then, may not cause neurological abnormalities unless the spinal canal is already narrowed developmentally. Sufficient reserve space should be available, especially since the cervical cord normally measures 8 mm in the sagittal plane by 13 mm in the transverse plane (48). Accordingly, patients with spondylotic myelopathy have an average lower cervical canal diameter which measures 3 mm less than those with spondylosis without myelopathy (3,52).

As in the case of lumbar spinal stenosis, the midline and lateral sagittal cervical canal diameter is determined by the height and vertical angle of the pedicles (20,34). The embryological basis for these variations is unknown. The position of the superior facet with respect to the vertebral body, as seen on lateral cervical spine radiographs, provides an indication of the pedicle height and canal diameter (34). Since the superior facet arises dorsally from the pedicle, and it is more easily visualized radiographically, observing its position in the anteroposterior (A-P) plane is useful in estimating the dimensions of the neural canal.

The intervertebral foramina may also vary in dimension on a developmental basis. Normally, they are 5 to 7.5 mm long, 5 to 6 mm wide, and 10 to 13 mm in sagittal diameter (21). Moderate shortening or lateral angulation of the pedicles may narrow the foramina without causing signficant midline canal stenosis. However, since cervical nerve roots measure only 3 to 4 mm in diameter, radiculopathy is rarely if ever seen in stenosis patients who do not have associated spondylosis.

Severe developmental cervical spinal stenosis as a primary cause of myelopathy is rare. It is an easily overlooked cause of progressive neurological deficit since observation of concurrent spondylosis on radiographs does not draw attention to the reduced neural canal diameter. Kessler (42) reported six cases in a retrospective review of 1,174 records of cervical arthritis or laminectomy patients at New York Hospital. Three had no significant degenerative changes, and the others had only small osteophytes. Three of these patients were under the age of 40 and one was 15. In our series of 42 decompressive cervical laminectomies at the University of Arizona Hospitals, there were seven cases in which stenosis was considered to be a more significant pathogenetic factor for myelopathy than spondylosis. This 16% incidence may reflect an increase of awareness and more frequent diagnosis of the problem. As in lumbar stenosis, a striking male preponderance is observed, although one of our patients was a 32-year-old female whose average canal diameter measured 12 mm (Fig. 1) (35,45,50).

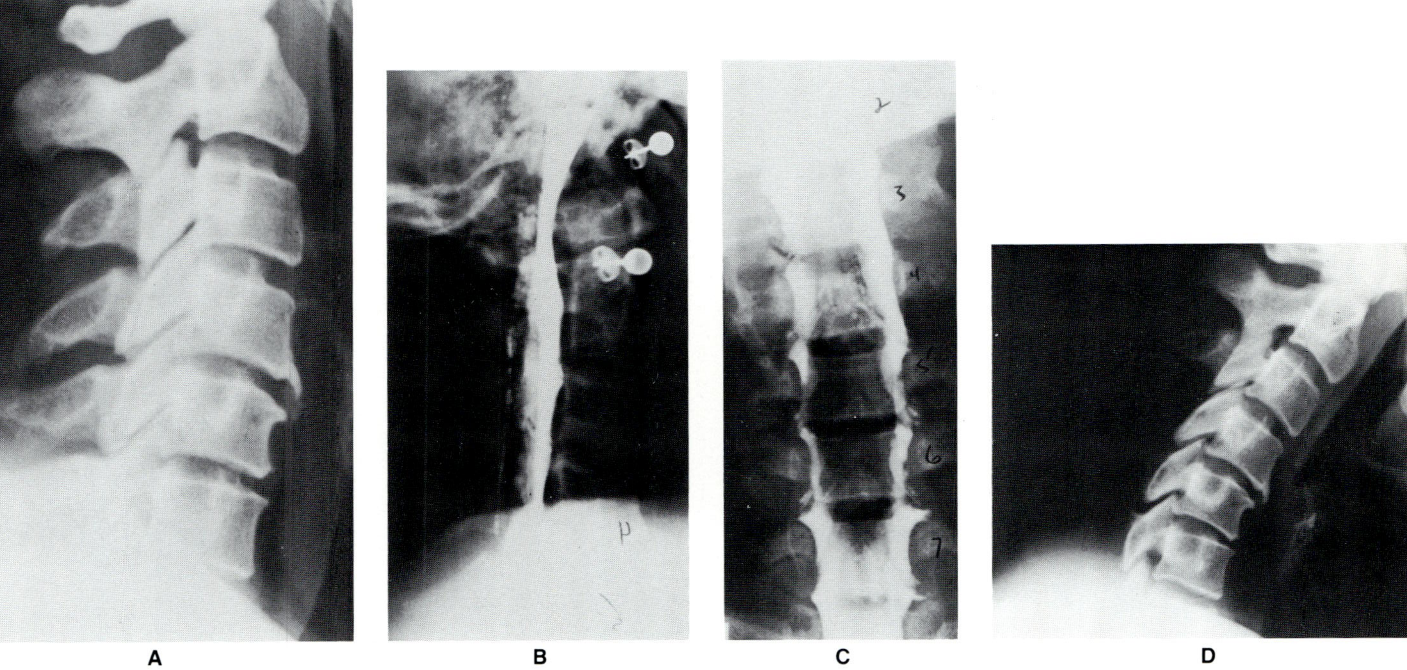

A B C D

FIG. 1. Cervical stenosis. **A:** Lateral radiograph in a 34-year-old female who presented with progressive weakness and activity-induced incoordination of the right hand, as well as early signs of myelopathy. She had bilateral extensor plantar responses with moderate gait spasticity and a sensory hypalgesia below T_3. Sagittal canal diameter measures 12 mm at C_4–C_5 and C_5–C_6. **B:** Lateral myelogram demonstrating smooth dorsal and ventral canal surfaces due to diffuse stenosis without spondylosis. **C:** Anteroposterior (AP) myelogram documenting cord compression with widening of the cord shadow at C_5 and C_6. **D:** Postoperative lateral radiograph in flexion showing maintainance of spinal stability after wide decompressive laminectomy at C_4–C_6. The patient recovered slowly over 4 months and returned to work as a supermarket cashier.

Associated congenital anomalies have been observed. The most common are the Klippel-Feil syndrome and other types of fused or block vertebrae (60). With anterior cervical fusion, we have recently treated successfully a patient with flexion-induced pain, Lhermitte's sign, and leg weakness, who had cervical stenosis and a congenital posterior fusion at C_3 to C_6 with anterior subluxation and spondylosis at C_2–C_3. Symptoms of pain and postural myelopathy were relieved without bothersome additional loss of cervical mobility by an anterior interbody fusion (Fig. 2).

The mechanism of premature embryological growth cessation which leads to spinal stenosis, with or without other anomalies, is unknown (19,42). Most postnatal growth of the cervical canal sagittal diameter occurs before the age of 3 since an average increase of only 3 mm is observed between the ages of 3 and 18 (36,42). Premature closure or fusion of paired neural arch and vertebral body ossification centers has been postulated as the cause of diffuse spinal stenosis in achondroplastic dwarfs (17). Such a mechanism could account for the shortened pedicles seen in developmental spinal stenosis.

Other conditions rarely associated with cervical spine stenosis include neurofibromatosis, osteopetrosis, spondyloepiphyseal dysplasia, pituitary gigantism, and Paget's disease (18,33,59,73). Bony overgrowth may result in myelopathy requiring laminectomy to relieve cord compression due to hypertrophic neural arches. After injury resulting in cervical fracture, disc rupture, or dislocation, localized post-traumatic spondylosis may also cause symptomatic spinal stenosis, especially if spinal deformity or vertebral subluxation persist. Idiopathic calcification or ossification of the posterolongitudinal ligament has also been observed in Japan and Western countries as a cause of cervical spinal stenosis and myelopathy (4,51,53).

Clinically, symptoms of cord compression are predominant, and neck pain or cervical radiculopathy are not severe or characteristic features in cervical stenosis patients. Neurological abnormalities do not differ from cases of spondylotic myelopathy. However, Kessler (42) found that sudden development of persistent myelopathy or brief transient episodes of myelopathic symptoms were both induced by increased physical activity in his series of cases. "Intermittent claudication" of the cervical spinal cord due to impaired or transiently inadequate blood flow was suggested as a possible explanation. Increased spinal cord metabolic rate during activity, loss of autoregulation of cord blood flow, and compression of arterial or venous channels have been proposed as contributing factors in patients with intermittent symptoms or acute onset of myelopathy (9,42,72).

FIG. 2. Spondylosis above congenital fusion with stenosis. **A:** Lateral radiograph in a 67-year-old man who presented with painful paresthesias on neck flexion and a normal neurological examination. An unusual form of probably congenital posterior fusion from C_3 to C_7 is noted with sagittal canal diameters of 13 to 17 mm. **B:** Flexion view demonstrating 5-mm anterior subluxation of C_2–C_3. No movement was observed at the lower segments. **C:** AP myelogram showing widening of the cord shadow. **D:** Lateral myelogram suggesting multilevel dorsal but not ventral stenosis to 8-mm sagittal diameter, which was not symptomatic and was not predicted from the plain film measurements. **E:** Postoperative lateral radiograph showing interbody bone graft at C_2 to C_3. All symptoms resolved after anterior fusion, and laminectomy was not performed.

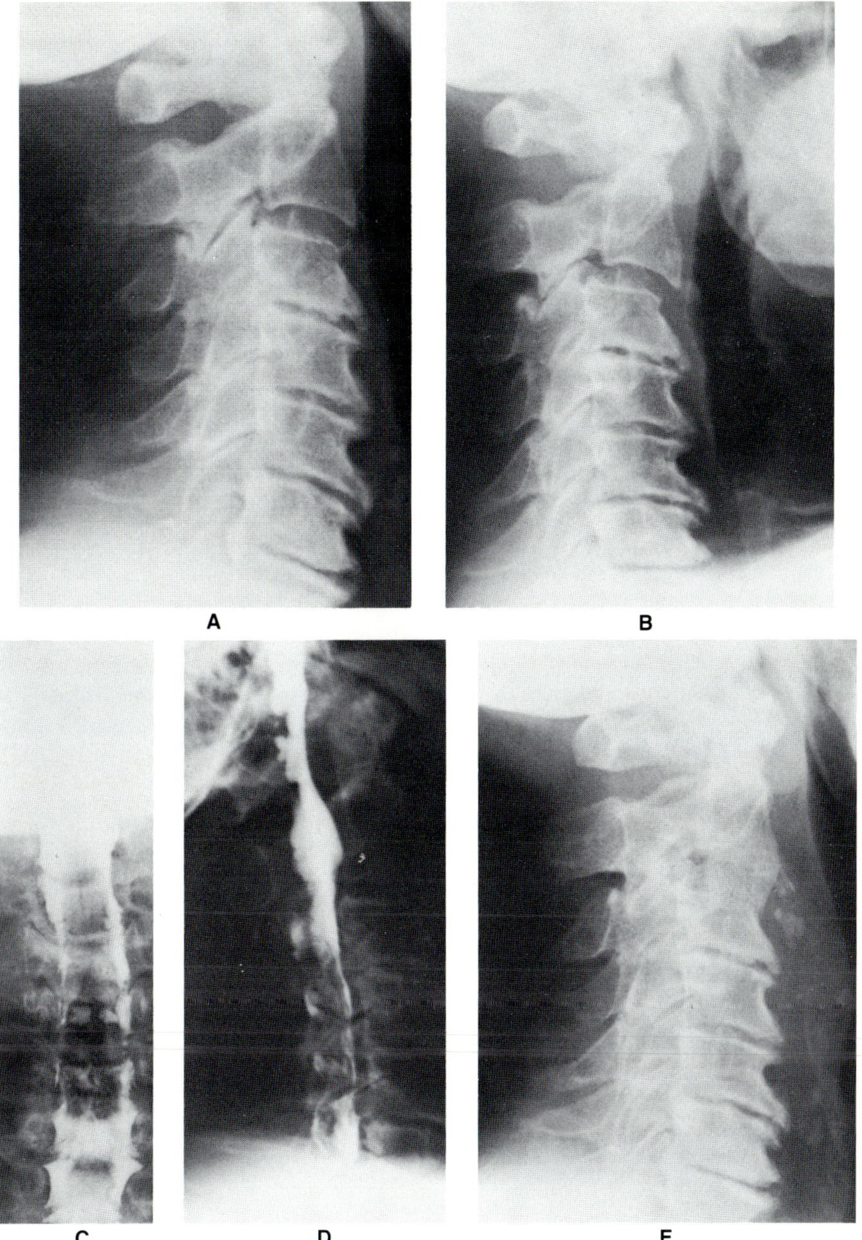

A   B

C   D   E

Spondylosis

The pathogenesis of cervical spondylosis has been described and illustrated clinically and pathologically (48,77). The primary event is intervertebral disc degeneration. As the nucleus dessicates after injury or with increasing age, the disc collapses. Attachment of the annulus to the vertebral body margin separates or tears, provoking a proliferative response. Reactive hyperplasia at the cartilaginous plate margin results in osteophyte formation and osteoneogenesis. Chronically herniated disc material and granulation tissue may also be incorporated in marginal osteophytes. The uncinate processes of cervical vertebral bodies are commonly involved sites of osteophyte formation which lie in the floor of the lateral recess of the neural canal anterior to emerging nerve roots as they enter their foramina.

Developmental regression or atheromatous degeneration of the circumferential arterial network supplying cervical vertebral bodies has also been implicated in the pathogenesis of osteophytosis and spondylotic osteomalacia (49). The role of trauma, stress, strain, and hypermobility in development of cervical spondylosis has also been studied (16). In addition to formation of ventral ridges which reduce the sagittal canal diameter, spondylosis is associated with posterior encroachment by hypertrophic ligamentum flavum which may thicken and buckle inward in association with disc collapse and spondylosis (19).

In addition to these well-known features of cervical spondylosis, the occurrence of degenerative spondylolisthesis and subluxation should be emphasized because of its role in producing stenosis and myelopathy (6). Anterolisthesis or retrolisthesis due to disc collapse and ligamentous laxity may be observed as a static deformity, or as a dynamic process developing during flexion or extension of the cervical spine. Failure to recognize degenerative cervical spondylolisthesis may result in progression, postoperatively, after anterior discectomy or laminectomy and foramenotomy, without concomitant fusion.

Since the cervical cord follows the shortest route through the spinal canal, as observed during experimental myelographic studies in cadavers, it may be drawn tightly against either the anterior or posterior surfaces of a stenotic neural canal. This is especially true if kyphotic or lordotic deformities develop due to spondylosis (6). Flexion of a kyphotic and spondylotic cervical spine may further stretch the cord over anterior osteophytes also causing compression of the anterior spinal artery.

Myelopathy

Myelopathy in cervical stenosis and spondylosis is primarily due to mechanical compression of the cord. Autopsy studies of untreated multilevel spondylosis patients with progression to quadriparesis show extensive distortion and destruction of the cord in both grey and white matter corresponding with the location of large ventral osteophytes in canals with a narrow sagittal diameter. Focal vascular thrombosis is observed (54,77). Extent of cord infarction correlates well with degree of spinal stenosis. Posterior column involvement was extensive and could have been predicted from impairment of touch, vibration, and joint position sense in advanced cases (54). Demyelination of involved ascending and descending tracts was observed above and below the cervical lesions. Pathological changes in the nerve roots include degeneration, atrophy, and periradicular fibrosis (26,32,54).

Experimental studies in a canine model of cervical myelopathy suggest that the effects of cord compression upon neurological function are probably mediated by alterations of blood flow (28,38). Microangiographic and autoradiography studies indicate that systemic hypotension and ligation of vertebral as well as anterior spinal and radicular arteries are synergistic with mechanical cord compression by 25% reduction of sagittal canal diameters in producing myelopathy and reducing cord blood flow (29,38,40). The effects of multilevel compression are also additive.

These results correspond with observations from the autopsy material (54). Thus one can surmise that transient, temporary, or permanent neurological deficit due to cervical cord compression may be caused by ischemia or infarction as well as direct constriction or deformation of neuroaxonal tissue.

CLINICAL FEATURES

Radiculopathy is by far the most common clinical manifestation of cervical spondylosis (7). Pain and sensory or motor deficit are more often chronic and gradual in onset than with radiculopathy due to soft disc extrusion. Severe spondylosis may be associated with either myelopathy alone, or myelopathy together with painful radiculopathy. Some of our most advanced cases of cord compression, however, complained of only mild neck discomfort. This may be explained by the observation that underlying cervical stenosis may reduce the sagittal canal diameter in the midline without narrowing lateral recesses or foramina (35). Conversely, patients with progressive myelopathy after surgical relief of radiculopathy by anterior or posterior foraminotomy may require a midline decompression for relief of previously unrecognized canal stenosis. We recently observed dramatic relief after reoperation by upper cervical laminectomy in a patient with severe quadriparesis who had remission of neck and arm pain, but not myelopathy, after C_5 to T_1 laminectomy 10 years previously, and anterior fusion at C_5 to C_7 7 years previously. Repeat myelography had demonstrated a complete block due to persistent stenosis at C_3 C_4.

Other controversial aspects of clinical diagnosis include occurrence of painless amyotrophy in the upper extremities which is not associated with a radicular sensory loss (14). Such deficits may be caused by ischemia or compression of the anterior horn neurons rather than their associated ventral roots. When concurrent lower extremity spasticity and corticospinal tract signs are present, the diagnosis of amyotrophic lateral sclerosis with incidental spondylosis is considered. In such patients, surgical decompression is recommended as a therapeutic trial only if myelography demonstrates a partial or complete block.

Correlation between the level of myelographic lesions and that of associated neurological deficit may be far from exact. In one of our recent cases, reversal of severely impaired fine motor coordination in the fingers of the left hand as well as gait spasticity, urinary frequency with incontinence, and extensor plantar responses followed laminectomy for stenosis and spondylosis at C_5 and C_6 (Fig. 3). Thus a myelopathic corticospinal tract lesion may be located two or more segments above the level of dysfunction, which in this case was not due to C_8 to T_1 radiculopathy. Similarly, we have observed C_6 myelopathy, presumably due to ischemia and spondylotic anterior spinal artery compression, resolve following anterior cervical decompression at C_3 to C_4.

Patients with severe stenosis and spondylosis are vulnerable to acute traumatic myelopathy. Relatively minor hyperextension injuries in this setting often result in severe deficit due to central cord contusion (66). Although immediate surgical decompression is known to aggravate rather than relieve such cord injuries, the presence of a sagittal canal diameter of 7 to 10 mm and a complete myelographic block justifies consideration of careful and meticulous surgical decompression, especially in patients who do not improve in 3 to 5 days after spinal immobilization and systemic administration of steroids. Thus, in our view, cervical stenosis patients

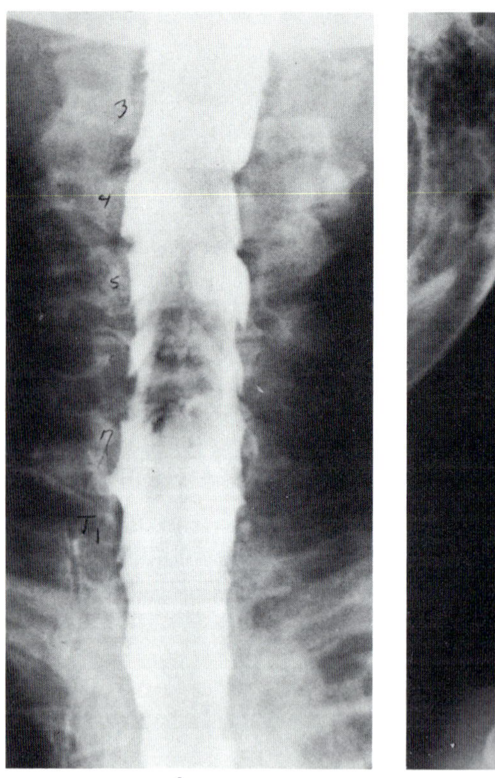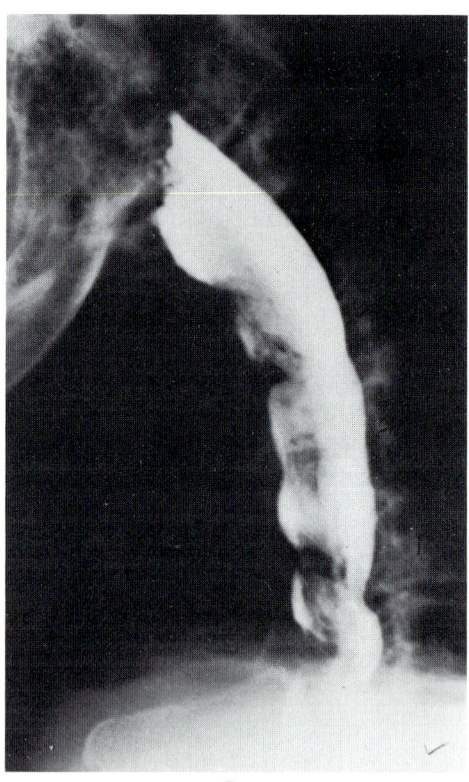

A   **B**

FIG. 3. Cervical myelopathy. **A:** AP myelogram in a 72-year-old woman with myelopathy, no evidence of radiculopathy, and loss of fine motor control of the left hand (see text). Note moderate thinning of contrast column at C_6. **B:** Lateral myelogram demonstrating ventral and dorsal defects at C_5–C_6 and C_6–C_7, two segments above the level of neurological impairment.

represent a special group of central cord contusion patients who may not always fit the criteria for nonoperative management. Recovery is unlikely if cord compression persists.

Recommendation of prophylactic surgical decompression to prevent recurrent or future cord damage from hyperextension injury in cervical stenosis patients remains controversial. Unless (a) dangerous instability due to degenerative spondylolisthesis is observed, (b) failure to fully recover from previous cord contusion occurs in the presence of a myelographic block, or (c) a progressive myelopathic syndrome develops, the risk of spinal surgery is difficult to justify.

RADIOLOGICAL DIAGNOSIS

Cervical spine radiographs should provide an accurate estimate of the sagittal diameter of the spinal canal and foramina. However, one must interpret oblique views cautiously since the degree of foraminal encroachment demonstrated may vary significantly with the angle of projection of the X-ray beam as determined by the degree of rotation of the spinal column. Lateral flexion-extension views should always be obtained so that the possibility of reduction of the static canal diameter by postural changes can be evaluated. In some spondylosis patients, dense articular sclerosis and eburnation, ligamentous ossification, and proliferative osteophyte formation may obliterate normal bony landmarks. Lateral tomograms will then be helpful to delineate the true sagittal diameter of the neural canal, lateral recesses, and foramina. When degenerative or traumatic spondylolisthesis or subluxation is present, obtaining routine tomography in addition to tomography during flexion and extension has been useful in the diagnosis of static or dynamic cervical stenosis.

Computed tomographic (CT) imaging of the cervical spine shows promise for providing an invaluable method of diagnosis of spinal stenosis (74). Especially since the development of thin section and preliminary scout film localizer techniques, segmental visualization of the cervical spinal column in axial or reconstructed sagittal sections has become routine in many medical centers. Sagittal and transverse canal dimensions can be easily measured (Fig. 4). However, although facet and laminar hypertrophy can be demonstrated consistently, osteophytes and herniated discs may not be visualized unless calcification or ossification has occurred. Thus, ligamentous hypertrophy or soft disc herniation can be missed unless displacement of an interface with the lower density epidural fat layer can be identified. Unless serial 5-mm sections are obtained, areas of focal stenosis due to facets or osteophytes may not be demonstrated.

Myelography remains the standard and most reliable method for diagnosing cervical stenosis and spondylosis. Lateral and frontal views obtained in the neutral and extended postures are also helpful for demonstrating dynamic factors influencing canal diameter and severity of cervical cord compression (20). The cord will appear flattened in the lateral projection and widened in the frontal projection when severe spinal stenosis is present (Fig. 1). If spondylosis contributes, typical ventral disc ridges and dorsal *ligamentum flavum* and facet indentations will be present, often

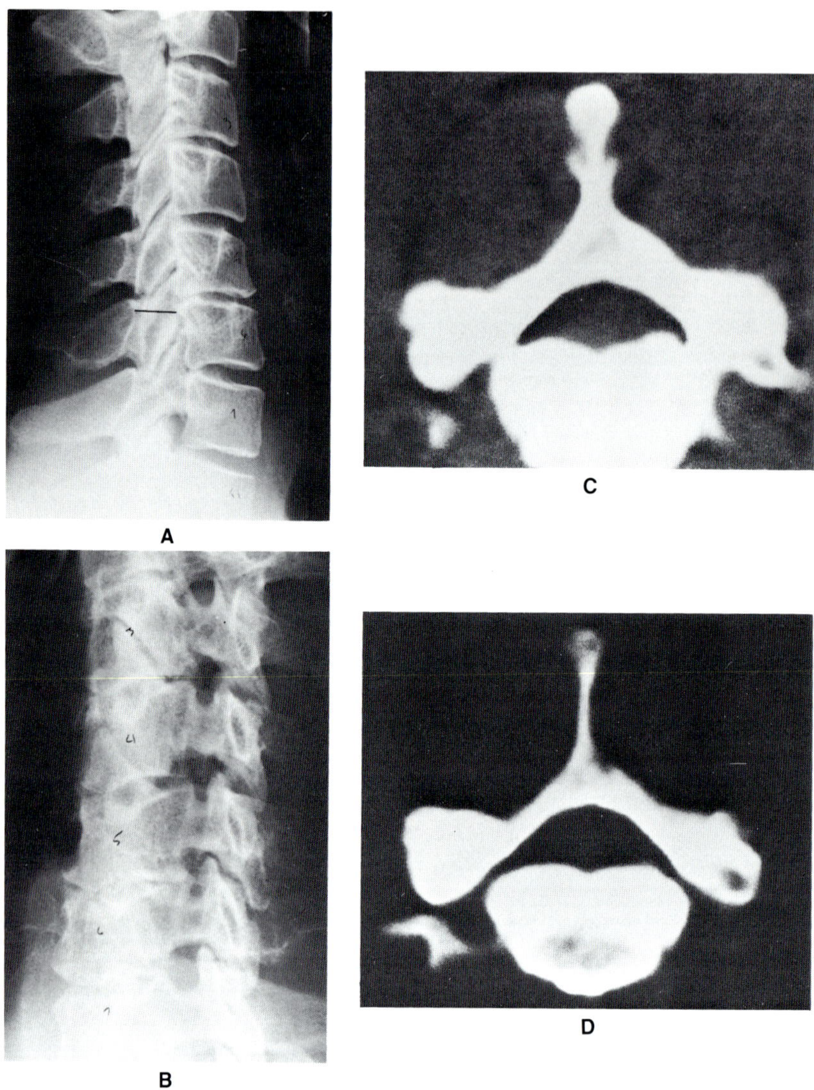

FIG. 4. Cervical radiculopathy. **A:** Lateral radiograph of a 50-year-old physician with a 12-year history of intermittent disabling bilateral C_6 radiculopathy. No evidence of myelopathy was found. Sagittal canal diameters average 12 mm *(dark line)*. **B:** Oblique radiograph demonstrating foraminal encroachment by an osteophyte at C_5–C_6 on the left. **C:** Coronal section with CT scanner, taken through the pedicles of C_5, demonstrating ventrolateral uncinate process hypertrophy and reduction of sagittal canal diameter to 10 mm. **D:** Lower section through the lateral recesses at C_5–C_6 showing marked foraminal stenosis with relatively less bony constriction in the midline. Myelography demonstrated a subtotal block at C_5–C_6 due to the ventral osteophyte without evidence of dorsal cord compression. Symptoms were relieved by anterior decompression without interbody fusion.

at multiple levels (Fig. 3). Such findings are considered to be unequivocal indications for surgical decompression when a partial or complete myelographic block is demonstrated which is not relieved by neck flexion.

At times, the true sagittal canal diameter may be difficult to estimate on the lateral myelogram because contrast material forms a thin undulating layer on the ventral surface. High volume iophendylate (Pantopaque®) or high concentration amipaque (Metrizimide®) injections may be necessary in order to accurately assess volume of the cervical subarachnoid space from the foramen magnum to the cervicothoracic junction. At present, myelography remains the optimum method for defining the longitudinal extent of cervical spine stenosis for purposes of planning the extent of required surgical decompression. As further experience is acquired, CT scanning may prove to be sufficient in the future.

SURGICAL THERAPY—CONTROVERSIES

Most of the controversies regarding treatment of cervical stenosis and spondylosis relate to indications for, and methods of, surgical decompression. A trial of conservative therapy with 10 to 14 days of bed rest followed by use of a firm cervical collar for 1 to 2 months is usually indicated. This is especially appropriate in elderly patients with diffuse spondylosis and minimal chronic cervical myelopathy. One may observe partial resolution of spasticity and disappearance of extensor plantar responses following partial immobilization of the cervical spine. All patients presenting with radiculopathy without myelopathy should be treated conservatively since many will improve without surgery. However, symptoms and signs of radiculopathy or myelopathy may recur when normal activity is resumed, and these patients must be followed closely with repeat neurological examinations. Theoretically, cervical spine traction or manipulation should be of no therapeutic value in patients with myelopathy caused by osteophytosis and compression due to cervical stenosis or severe spondylosis. Occasionally, traction may relieve radiculopathy patients.

On the other hand, patients with documented progression of moderate or severe cervical myelopathy are unlikely to improve with any form of conservative treatment. Especially when intermittent symptoms of "cord claudication" or episodes of abrupt onset of cord dysfunction suggest vascular compromise in patients with cervical stenosis, myelography should be performed and surgical decompression advised.

If myelographic findings are equivocal and the diagnosis is unclear, or if a neuroaxonal degenerative disease is suspected, surgery should be deferred. If under observation, progression of myelopathy with more precise neurological localization and myelographic correlation is documented, the indications for surgical decompression are better established. Since irreversible damage from cord compression or infarction may have already occurred, patients are advised that the goal of surgery is primarily to prevent further neurological deterioration (38). Although recovery of motor and sensory deficits due to cervical radiculopathy is commonly observed in 80 to 100% of patients, improvement in myelopathy occurs in only 50 to 70% and is unpredictable—especially in advanced cases (6,12,24,30,44,65,70).

Indications for prophylactic decompression or fusion in asymptomatic cervical stenosis patients and those with a history of pain or minor trauma without neurological deficit remain controversial. Information from a prospective study of the natural history of patients with developmental, traumatic, or spondylotic narrowing of the cervical canal would be required to make a scientific decision in this regard. Fortunately, this question does not arise too often. When it does, it has not been our policy to advise decompressive surgery for asymptomatic stenosis even when sagittal canal diameters measure less than 12 mm. However, when traumatic or degenerative subluxation as demonstrated on flexion-extension views reduces the sagittal canal diameter to 10 mm or less, fusion with anterior or posterior decompression is indicated. Surgery should be advised, prophylactically, especially if pain and neurological deficits are elicited by extremes of cervical spine movement. In addition, patients with severe stenosis who recover from cervical cord contusion should be considered for surgical decompression to prevent recurrent cord injury even if spinal instability is not observed.

Selection of the anterior or posterior surgical procedure for myelopathy depends upon the anatomy of each individual patient's disease. The anterolateral approach for removal of osteophytes has also been described (75). This decision should not be based only on the surgeon's personal preference or the results of large retrospective clinical surveys which do not stratify analysis of such variables as sagittal bony canal diameter, number of levels involved, and the relative contributions to stenosis of anterior osteophytes, posterior ligaments, or degenerative spondylolisthesis. Patients with developmental cervical spinal stenosis and sagittal canal diameters of less than 12 mm because of short pedicles are certainly best treated by wide laminectomy rather than anterior fusion over all involved levels (15). Cases of severe spondylosis with small 1 to 2 mm anterior bar discs and large posterior ligamentous and laminar or facet indentations seen myelographically should also undergo a posterior rather than anterior decompression. When significant 3 to 4 mm degenerative or traumatic spondylolisthesis is observed, fusion should be added by the posterolateral or anterior interbody techniques, depending upon which approach has been selected as most appropriate for decompression. If large 2 to 4 mm anterior osteophytes are present in patients with minimal posterior myelographic defects, and sagittal canal diameters are adequate above and below the osteophytes, anterior discectomy may be the procedure of choice. This removes the pathological structures compressing the cord and its vasculature rather than allowing the cord to move away from the pathology as would be the case with laminectomy. Results may be slightly better after anterior fusion than laminectomy in myelopathy patients (30).

In some spondylotic myelopathy cases, equally large anterior and posterior myelographic abnormalities are seen without evidence of severe developmental stenosis. Here either anterior or posterior decompression is appropriate. At times both procedures may be necessary if the patient continues to deteriorate or fails to improve after the primary operation (47). Repeat myelography should be obtained, however, in order to confirm the persistence of cord compression.

The longitudinal extent of decompressive surgery for myelopathy should depend more on the myelogram and CT scan than neurological localization of myelopathy. We decompress all myelographically stenotic levels assuming that persistent cord compression at unoperated levels may produce symptoms and signs in the future. This, of course, is not the case in decompressive surgery for cervical radiculopathy which should be limited to levels which correlate with clear signs of nerve root dysfunction. If the anterior approach is selected, and more than two or three levels require discectomy or fusion, the operation can be performed in two or more stages. However, many surgeons prefer decompressive laminectomy for treatment of myelopathy due to three or four level spondylosis. Under these circumstances, the posterior approach offers the advantage of completing the necessary decompression in one operation without the disadvantages of resulting multiple-level arthrodesis following bone graft or simple discectomy.

Adequate posterior decompression, especially for myelopathy due to cervical stenosis, requires wide laminectomy, and even medial facetectomy, in order to fully unroof the spinal canal and lateral recesses (6,70). Foraminotomy may be indicated at some levels, and on one or both sides selected by clinical and myelographic findings in those rare patients who suffer from radiculopathy as well as myelopathy (24,67). However, radical bilateral foraminotomy or facetectomy may in a small number of cases lead to postoperative instability and subluxation causing recurrent symptoms (47). Reoperation for anterior or posterior fusion may be necessary.

Excision of osteophytes with angled down-biting curettes and osteotomes has been recommended for completion of posterior decompression of both myelopathy and radiculopathy (22,24). Improvement was observed in 80% of patients so treated, as compared to 50% in those treated by posterior decompression alone (22). In our experience, and in that of others, this maneuver has not been necessary unless inspection reveals persistent posterior displacement of the dura or nerve roots of more than 3 to 4 mm by osteophytes or chronically herniated disc material (6).

Although the sitting position has been advocated for posterior cervical decompression, we strongly recommend the prone position for all myelopathy patients, despite the minor inconvenience of increased intraoperative venous bleeding (24,67). Since impairment of spinal cord blood flow and its autoregulation have been identified experimentally as factors contributing to compressive myelopathy, the increased risk of intraoperative hypotension and air embolism in the sitting position should be avoided (28,55).

Another unresolved controversy persists with respect to whether or not section of the dentate ligaments is beneficial (24). Tethering of the spinal cord to the anterior surface of the canal has been suggested and documented by gas myelography in some cases (13,41). Experimental studies in a canine model showed that reduction of somatosensory evoked potentials produced by elevation of the cord upon nylon slings was eliminated by section of the dentate ligaments (13). Human cadaver studies have also documented reduction in force required to elevate the cord with the spine flexed after dentate section (9,13). However, others have questioned the significance of these observations showing little influence of dentate section upon posterior migration of the cord in cadaver studies (61,68). Adequate posterior transposition of the cord has also been observed during postoperative myelography in patients decompressed without dentate section (1). Moreover, some clinical studies show little additional benefit from dentate resection in myelopathy patients (30,58). Accordingly, dentate ligament section should perhaps be considered only if anterior tethering of the cord can be documented by gas or amipaque myelography or CT spine scan in those few patients who fail to improve after decompressive laminectomy.

Durotomy and closure with a dural graft has also not been routinely necessary in our experience. Only in occasional cases of severe congenital stenosis or chronic post-traumatic dislocation has the dural sac failed to expand adequately following bony decompression. However, when extensive epidural scarring, circumferential dural thickening, or a persistently tight dural sac is observed, longitudinal incision and closure with an elliptical graft of fascia or dural substitute will be necessary to relieve cord compression.

The controversy as to whether or not bone grafting is preferable or beneficial following anterior discectomy and foraminotomy for spondylosis is unsettled (46). Resorption of osteophytes after cervical interbody fusion without excision of osteophytes has been documented by postoperative radiographs and myelography (5,63,64). However, occurrence of spondylosis at levels above or below the surgical fusion has also been documented and raised as a consideration in addition to decreased surgical morbidity in favor of simple microsurgical osteophyte excision and foraminotomy by the anterior approach without bone grafting (8,39). However, spontaneous fusion will occur eventually in most cases after discectomy alone (62,78). One advantage of bone graft fusion which may be important in selected cases is that distraction of the interspace with bone grafts is observed to reduce posterior myelographic defects because of infolding of the ligamentum flavum (5). Elimination of motion and minor recurrent cord injury at the spondylotic or stenotic interspace, however, can be achieved in most cases with either technique since discectomy alone ultimately results in spontaneous interbody fusion (44).

Use of the operating microscope for anterior surgical decompression is no longer controversial since it clearly allows more accurate and safer removal of disc and osteophytes with limited enlargement of the interspace (39,43). Thus bone graft fusion may be unnecessary since stability is retained and height of the adjacent bodies is preserved.

Complete removal of the posterior longitudinal ligament, which may increase intraoperative bleeding and postoperative instability, is rarely necessary for adequate decompression, although detachment from vertebral body margins and osteophytes is essential. Inspection of the epidural space through a small incision in the ligament is recommended in cases where an extruded disc fragment is suspected or the ligament is hypertrophic.

Postoperative flexion deformity or progression of subluxation has not been observed in our experience with anterior discectomy and decompression for spondylosis, even when 1 to 2 mm preoperative degenerative spondylolisthesis is present, if no additional movement is seen on flexion-extension radiographs. However, when more extensive subluxation is observed preoperatively, or the presence of a well-maintained disc space suggests that discectomy and collapse of the interspace might aggravate foramenal encroachment postoperatively despite osteophyte excision, interbody bone graft fusion may be indicated. Our standard anterior procedure for spondylosis, except in these unusual circumstances, is microsurgical interbody decompression without fusion.

The question of degree and duration of clinical improvement, and incidence of postoperative neurological complications after laminectomy for stenosis, and anterior or posterior decompression for spondylosis, can only be answered by long-term follow-up studies (2,12,30,31). In our experience, immediate postoperative neurological deterioration has been temporary in all but two of 46 myelopathy patients. All three primary developmental stenosis patients in our series improved significantly, but not completely, after laminectomy.

SUMMARY

On the basis of current knowledge of the anatomy and pathophysiology of the cervical spine, cord, and nerve roots, as well as recent diagnostic advances such as CT spine scanning, surgical therapy can be recommended and planned in a more rational manner. Determination of the extent of decompression and selection of a surgical approach should be decided individually in each case depending upon a detailed analysis of radiographic studies.[1] In this manner, resolution of some of the controversies in this field may yield improvement in clinical results.

REFERENCES

1. Aboulker, J., David, M., Engel, P., and Ballivet, J. (1965): Les myelopathies cervicales d'origine rachidienne. *Neurochirurgie*, 11:87–198.
2. Adams, C. (1976): Cervical spondylotic radiculopathy and myelopathy. *Handbook of Clin. Neurol.*, 26:97–112.
3. Arnold, J. G. (1955): The clinical manifestations of spondylochondrosis (spondylosis) of the cervical spine. *Ann. Surg.*, 141:872–889.
4. Bakay, L., Cares, H. L., and Smith, R. J. (1970): Ossification in the region of the posterior longitudinal ligament as a cause of cervical myelopathy. *J. Neurol. Neurosurg. Psychiat.*, 33:263.
5. Bohlman, H. H. (1977): Cervical spondylosis with moderate to severe myelopathy. A report of seventeen cases treated by Robinson anterior cervical discectomy and fusion. *Spine*, 2:151–162.
6. Braakman, R. (1979): Cervical spondylotic myelopathy. In: *Advances and Technical Standards in Neurosurgery*, Vol. 6. Edited by H. Krayenbuhl, pp. 137–169. Springer-Verlag, New York.

---

[1]Perhaps future developments such as use of intraoperative monitoring of somatosensory or vestibular spinal evoked potentials will render decompressive surgery safer and more accurate.

7. Brain, W. R., Northfield, D., Wilkinson, M. (1952): The neurological manifestations of cervical spondylosis. *Brain,* 75:187–225.
8. Braunstein, E. M., Hunter, L. Y., Bailey, R. W. (1980): Long term radiographic changes following anterior cervical fusion. *Clin. Radiol.,* 31:201–203.
9. Breig, A., Turnbull, I., Hassler, O. (1966): Effects of mechanical stresses on the spinal cord in cervical spondylosis. A study on fresh cadaver material. *J. Neurosurg.,* 25:45–56.
10. Brooker, A. E. W., Barter, R. W. (1965): Cervical spondylosis: A clinical study with comparative radiology. *Brain,* 88:925–936.
11. Burrows, E. H. (1963): The sagittal diameter of the spinal canal in cervical spondylosis. *Clin. Radiol.,* 17:77–86.
12. Crandall, P. H., Gregorius, F. K. (1977): Long-term follow-up of surgical treatment of cervical spondylotic myelopathy. *Spine,* 2:139–146.
13. Cusick, J. F., Ackmann, J. J., Larson, S. J. (1977): Mechanical and physiological effects of dentatomy. *J. Neurosurg.,* 46:767–775.
14. Dorsen, M., Ehni, G. (1979): Cervical spondylotic radiculopathy producing motor manifestations mimicking primary muscular atrophy. *Neurosurg.,* 5:427–431.
15. Dunsker, S. B. (1976): Anterior cervical discectomy with and without fusion. *Clin. Neurosurg.,* 24:516.
16. Dunsker, S. B., Colley, D. P., Mayfield, F. H. (1978): Kinematics of the cervical spine. *Clin. Neurosurg.,* 25:174–183.
17. Duvoisin, R. C., Yahr, M. D. (1962): Compressive spinal cord and root syndromes in achondroplastic dwarfs. *Neurol.,* 12:202–207.
18. Efird, T. A., Genant, H. K., Wilson, C. B. (1980): Pituitary gigantism with cervical spinal stenosis. *Amer. J. Roentgenol.,* 134:171–173.
19. Ehrenhaft, J. L. (1943): Development of the vertebral column as related to certain congenital and pathological changes. *Surg. Gynecol. Obstet.,* 76:282–292.
20. Epstein, B. S., Epstein, J. A., Jones, M. D. (1977): Cervical spinal stenosis. *Radiol. Clin. North Am.,* 15:215–226.
21. Epstein, B. S., Epstein, J. A., Jones, M. D. (1978): Anatomicoradiological correlations in cervical spine discal disease and stenosis. *Clin. Neurosurg.,* 25:148–173.
22. Epstein, J. A., Carras, R., Lavine, L. S., Epstein, B. S. (1969): The importance of removing osteophytes as part of the surgical treatment of myeloradiculopathy in cervical spondylosis. *J. Neurosurg.,* 30:219–226.
23. Epstein, J. A., Epstein, B. S., Lavine, L. S. (1963): Cervical spondylotic myelopathy. *Arch. Neurol.,* 3:307–317.
24. Fager, C. A. (1976): Rationale and techniques of posterior approaches to cervical disk lesions and spondylosis. *Surg. Clin. North Am.,* 56:581–592.
25. Friedenberg, Z. B., Miller, W. T. (1963): Degenerative disc disease of the cervical spine. *J. Bone Joint Surg.,* 45A:1171–1178.
26. Frykholm, R. (1951): Cervical nerve root compression resulting from disc degeneration and root sleeve fibrosis. *Acta Chir. Scand. (Suppl.),* 160:1–149.
27. Galera, R., Tovi, D. (1968): Anterior disc excision with interbody fusion in cervical spondylotic myelopathy and rhizopathy. *J. Neurosurg.,* 28:305–310.
28. Gooding, M. R., Wilson, C. B., Hoff, J. T. (1975): Experimental cervical myelopathy: Effects of ischemia and compression of the canine cervical spinal cord. *J. Neurosurg.,* 43:9–17.
29. Gooding, M. R., Wilson, C. B., Hoff, J. T. (1976): Experimental cervical myelopathy: Autoradiographic studies of spinal cord blood flow patterns. *Surg. Neurol.,* 5:233–239.
30. Gorter, K. (1976): Influence of laminectomy effect on the course of cervical myelopathy. *Acta Neurochir.,* 33:265.
31. Guidetti, B., Fortuna, A. (1969): Long-term results of surgical treatment of myelopathy due to cervical spondylosis. *J. Neurosurg.,* 30:714–721.
32. Hadley, L. A. (1976): *Roentgenographic Studies of the Spine,* 3rd ed., pp. 422–477. Charles C Thomas, Springfield, Illinois.
33. Hartman, J. T., Dohnm, D. F. (1966): Paget's disease of the spine with cord or nerve-root compression. Report of six cases. *J. Bone Joint Surg.,* 48A:1079–1084.
34. Hayashi, K., Tabuchi, K., Yabuki, T., Kurokawa, T., Seki, H. (1977): The position of the superior articular process of the cervical spine. Its relationship to cervical spondylotic radiculopathy. *Radiology,* 124:501–503.

35. Hinck, V. C., Gordy, P. D., Storino, H. E. (1966): Developmental stenosis of the cervical spinal canal. *Neurol.*, 14:864–868.
36. Hinck, V. C., Hopkins, C. E., Savara, B. S. (1962): Sagittal diameter of the cervical spinal in children. *Radiology*, 79:97–108.
37. Hinck, V. C., Sachdev, N. S. (1966): Developmental stenosis of the cervical spinal canal. *Brain*, 89:27–36.
38. Hoff, J., Nishimura, B. S., Pitts, L., Vilnis, V., Tuerk, K., Lagger, R. (1977): The role of ischemia in the pathogenesis of cervical spondylotic myelopathy. A review and new microangiographic evidence. *Spine*, 2:100–108.
39. Hoff, J. T., Wilson, C. B. (1979): Microsurgical approach to the anterior cervical spine and spinal cord. *Clin. Neurosurg.*, 26:513–528.
40. Hukuda, S., Wilson, C. B. (1972): Experimental cervical myelopathy: Effects of compression and ischemia on the canine cervical cord. *J. Neurosurg.*, 37:631–652.
41. Kahn, E. A. (1947): The role of the dentate ligaments in spinal cord compression and the syndrome of lateral sclerosis. *J. Neurosurg.*, 4:191–199.
42. Kessler, J. T. (1975): Congenital narrowing of the cervical spinal canal. *J. Neurol.*, 38:1218–1224.
43. Kosary, I. Z., Braham, J., Shacked, I., Shacked, R. Microsurgery in anterior approach to cervical discs. *Surg. Neurol.*, 6:275–277.
44. Lunsford, L. D., Bissonette, D. J., Zorub, D. S. (1980): Anterior surgery for cervical disc disease, Part 2: Treatment of cervical spondylotic myelopathy in 32 cases. *J. Neurosurg.*, 53:12–19.
45. Lurati, M., Mertens, H. G. (1971): Die Bedeutung der anlagebedingten enge des cervicalkanals für die cervicale myelopathie. *Z. Neurol.*, 199:46–66.
46. Martins, A. N. (1976): Anterior cervical discectomy with and without interbody bone graft. *J. Neurosurg.*, 44:290.
47. Mayfield, F. H. (1965*a*): Cervical spondylosis: A comparison of the anterior and posterior approaches. *Clin. Neurosurg.*, 13:181–188.
48. Mayfield, F. H. (1965*b*): Cervical spondylosis. Observations based on surgical treatment of 400 patients. *Postgrad. Med.*, 38:345–357.
49. Mayfield, F. H. (1979): Cervical spondylotic radiculopathy and myelopathy. *Adv. Neurol.*, 22:307–321.
50. Moiel, B. H., Raso, E., Waltz, T. A. (1970): Central cord syndrome resulting from congenital narrowness of the cervical spinal cord. *J. Trauma*, 10:502–510.
51. Nagashima, C. (1972): Cervical myelopathy due to ossification of the posterior longitudinal ligament. *J. Neurosurg.*, 37:653.
52. Nurick, S. (1972): The pathogenesis of the spinal cord disorder associated with cervical spondylosis. *Brain*, 95:87–100.
53. Ono, K., Ota, H., Tada, K., Hamada, H., Takaoka, K. (1977): Ossified posterior longitudinal ligament: A clinicopathological study. *Spine*, 2:126–138.
54. Ono, K., Ota, K., Yamamoto, T. (1977): Cervical myelopathy secondary to multiple spondylotic protrusions. A clinicopathologic study. *Spine*, 2:109–125.
55. Palleske, H. (1969): Experimental investigations on the regulations of the spinal cord circulation. *Acta Neurochir. (Wien)*, 21:319–326.
56. Payne, E. E., Spillane, J. D. (1957): The cervical spine: An anatomicropathological study of 70 specimens (using a special technique) with particular reference to the problem of cervical spondylosis. *Brain*, 80:571–596.
57. Penning, L. (1968): *Functional Pathology of the Cervical Spine.* Excerpta Medica, Amsterdam.
58. Piepgras, D. G. (1976): Posterior decompression for myelopathy due to cervical spondylosis: Laminectomy alone versus laminectomy with dentate ligament section. *Clin. Neurosurg.*, 24:508.
59. Post, M. J. D. (1980): Computed tomography of the spine: Its values and limitations on a nonhigh resolution scanner. In: *Radiographic Evaluation of the Spine. Current Advances with Emphasis on Computed Tomography*, edited by M. J. D. Post, pp. 186–294. Masson Publishing Co., New York.
60. Ramsey, J., Bliznack, J. (1971): Klippel-Feil syndrome with renal agenesis and other anomalies. *Amer. J. Roentgenol.*, 113:460.
61. Reid, J. D. (1960): Ascending nerve roots and tightness of dura mater. a) Ascending nerve roots, b) Effects of flexion-extension movements of the head and spine upon the spinal cord and nerve roots. *J. Neurol. Neurosurg. Psychiatry*, 23:148–155, 214–221.

62. Robertson, J. T. (1973): Anterior removal of cervical disc without fusion. *Clin. Neurosurg.*, 20:259.
63. Robinson, R. A., Afeiche, N., Dunn, E. J., Northrup, B. E. (1977): Cervical spondylotic myelopathy. Etiology and treatment concepts. *Spine*, 2:89–99.
64. Robinson, R. A., Walker, A. E., Ferlie, D. C., Wiecking, D. K. (1962): The results of anterior interbody fusion of the cervical spine. *J. Bone Joint Surg.*, 44A:1569–1587.
65. Saunders, R. L., Wilson, D. H. (1980): The surgery of cervical disk disease: New perspectives. *Clin. Orthop. Rel. Res.*, 146:119–127.
66. Schneider, R. C., Cherry, G., Pantnek, H. (1954): The syndrome of acute central cervical spinal cord injury with special reference to the mechanisms involved in hyperextension injuries of the cervical spine. *J. Neurosurg.*, 11:546–577.
67. Scoville, W. B. (1961): Cervical spondylosis treated by bilateral facectomy and laminectomy. *J. Neurosurg.*, 18:423–428.
68. Stoltman, H. F. (1966): An anatomical study of the role of the dentate ligaments in the cervical spinal canal. *J. Neurosurg.*, 24:43–46.
69. Stoltman, H. F., Blackwood, W. (1964): The role of the ligamenta flava in the pathogenesis of myelopathy in cervical spondylosis. *Brain*, 87:45–50.
70. Stoops, W. L., King, R. B. (1965): Chronic myelopathy associated with cervical spondylosis—its response to laminectomy and foraminotomy. *J.A.M.A.*, 192:281–284.
71. Symon, L. Lavender, P. (1967): The surgical treatment of cervical spondylotic myelopathy. *Neurol.*, 17:117–127.
72. Turnbull, I. M. (1973): Blood supply of the spinal cord: Normal and pathological considerations. *Clin. Neurosurg.*, 20:56–84.
73. Vancoillie, P., Veiga-Pires, J. A. (1979): Cervical neurofibroma and generalised spinal stenosis in von Recklinghausen's disease. *Lancet*, 8154:1246–1247.
74. Verbiest, H. (1980): The value of CT-scan of the spine to the neurosurgeon. In: *Radiographic Evaluation of the Spine: Current Advances with Emphasis on Computed Tomography*, edited by M. J. D. Post, pp. 139–185. Masson Publishing Co., New York.
75. Verbiest, H., Geuse, H. D. (1966): Anterolateral surgery for cervical spondylosis in cases of myelopathy or nerve-root compression. *J. Neurosurg.*, 25:611–622.
76. Wilkinson, H. A., Le May, M. L., Ferris, E. J. (1969): Roentgenographic correlations in cervical spondylosis. *Amer. J. Roentgenol.*, 105:370–374.
77. Wilkinson, M. (1971): *Cervical Spondylosis. Its Early Diagnosis and Treatment*, edited by M. Wilkinson. W. B. Saunders Co., Philadelphia.
78. Wilson, D. H., Campbell, D. D. (1977): Anterior cervical discectomy without bone graft (report of 71 cases). *J. Neurosurg.*, 47:551.
79. Wolf, B. S., Khilnani, M., Malis, L. (1956): The sagittal diameter of the bony cervical spinal canal and its significance in cervical spondylosis. *J. Mt. Sinai Hosp.*, 23:283–292.

Controversies in Neurology, edited by R. A. Thompson and J. R. Green. Raven Press, New York © 1983.

Surgical Approach to Cervical Disc Disease With and Without Fusion

James T. Robertson

Department of Neurosurgery, The University of Tennessee Center for the Health Sciences, Memphis, Tennessee 38163

The anterior approach to the cervical spine for treatment of the various manifestations of cervical disc disease is the most common surgical approach used by neurosurgeons. This striking departure from the posterior approach is emphasized by review of the experiences of the neurosurgeons being examined by the American Board of Neurological Surgery. The advantages of the procedure are reduced patient morbidity, ease of performance with minimal blood loss, earlier discharge date, and, when the microscope is not used in the posterior approach, reduced nerve root trauma during the operation.

Bailey and Bagley (1) of Michigan were the first to describe the anterior approach to the cervical spine with fusion. They recommended a trough-onlay fusion for stabilizing traumatic and postsurgical dislocations and destructive vertebral lesions. The procedure was first performed in 1952 and consists of a trough cut into the anterior aspect of the vertebral bodies about ½ inch wide and 3/16 of an inch deep. The cut is through the full vertical height of the vertebrae. The discs are removed by the ronguer to a depth of 3/16 of an inch, and the cartilaginous plates on the inferior and superior aspects of the vertebral bodies are removed. The bone graft is put in place and the prevertebral fascia is resutured over it to maintain it in position. After this procedure, it is necessary to maintain the patient in traction for 6 weeks followed by bracing until satisfactory fusion occurs.

Smith and Robinson (21), in 1955, developed the anterior approach to the cervical spine with interbody fusion for the treatment of cervical disc disease and myelopathy. After initial animal experience, the technique was applied clinically. The anterior spine was approached through a vertical incision in the left anterolateral neck, and, after the removal of most of the degenerative disc material under direct vision, the vertebral bodies were separated as widely as the ligaments would allow, and a block of bone was placed in the intervertebral space. This procedure was thought to halt spur formation, relieve nerve root compression, and stop motion. In their initial report, they removed only the degenerate disc material within the interspace, allowing the remaining material in the spinal canal to be removed by "cellular activity." Shortly thereafter, Cloward (3,4) introduced the dowel interbody graft technique. Through his publications and speaking efforts, he, more than any other individual, stimulated the present enthusiasm for the approach to the anterior cervical spine. Initially, this technique was criticized by the senior neurosurgeons. Mayfield (10) modified the Smith-Robinson interbody fusion plug technique.

In 1969, Simmons and Bhalla (20) reported and described a keystone graft for interbody fusion. They did an excellent study on contrasting the various mechanical and clinical considerations of the dowel versus the keystone graft. The surface area of a bone graft does have important relationships to revascularization and bony union. The surface area of the rectangular graft is approximately 30% more than the surface area of the cylindrical graft. In addition, stability studies showed the keystone graft was more stable than the dowel graft and, finally, the fusion rate was 100% with the keystone graft.

Meanwhile, Hirsch (7), in 1960, described the first partial removal of a cervical disc by the anterior approach without interbody fusion. He used a vertical skin incision, and after incising the anterior longitudinal ligament and annulus, the disc was curetted to a varying degree and removed. The cartilaginous plates and opposing vertebral surfaces were not removed unless the interspace was narrowed markedly, and then only a partial removal was effected. Seventy percent of his patients were improved. None had an unstable spine, and bony fusion occurred in some of the cases. Hirsch raised the question as to how partial disc resection could eliminate the patient's symptoms. Although I am unable to answer this, it would appear that the results of his operation did not depend on the amount of disc material removed. He noted for the first time, without explanation, that occasionally a patient would develop distressing pain in the opposite extremity 2 to 3 weeks after the operation. He made no effort to remove all of the posterior annulus and apparently never interrupted the posterior longitudinal ligament or removed osteophytes.

Boldrey (2), in 1964, described the partial anterior removal of cervical discs without fusion with satisfactory results. Susen (22) presented excellent results with simple anterior cervical disc removal without fusion in 1966. He, like Boldrey, made no attempt to remove the cartilaginous plate or the entire disc.

Murphy and Gado (12) reported excellent results with disc removal alone in 26 patients with soft lateral extruded cervical discs. The disc removal was partial, without any special effort to remove the posterior osteophytes or the cartilaginous plate. They reported a 72% incidence of fusion following this procedure at one level. They confirmed that even in cases where incomplete X-ray fusion occurred, stability was present. Additionally, 50% of their cases showed resorption to some degree of the posterior osteophytes after 12 months. Thus, the presence or absence of a solid fusion did not effect the clinical result. This resorption of the posterior osteophytes compares favorably with resorption following interbody fusion as reported by Robinson (18), and DePalma and Rothman (5). The incidence of 72% solid fusion with partial disc removal was slightly less than the authors reported using interbody bone graft procedures.

In 1971, this author's series comparing anterior cervical disc treated with and without interbody fusion using the Cloward technique was reported to the American Academy of Neurological Surgery (14). The results were superior with simple discectomy. The anterior cervical spine was exposed as described by Cloward with wide incision and excision of the anterior longitudinal ligament and annulus of the disc followed by thorough curettement of all the disc material that could be removed including the cartilaginous plates. Using the operating microscope, the hole in the annulus through which the disc had ruptured was usually identified. Subsequently, the posterior annulus was either completely removed with or without removal of all or a portion of the posterior longitudinal ligament. The result did not appear to effect whether or not the entire posterior annulus and posterior longitudinal ligament were completely interrupted. The microscope was of great benefit in performing the procedure as well as appreciating the pathology. Use of the microscope was reemphasized in a publication by Hankinson and Wilson (6). They reported a series of cases treated by anterior disc removal without fusion although using a slightly different technique. They make an opening in the annulus and interspace in a central position no wider than 10 mm with columns of disc preserved on both sides. Using the operating microscope and air turbine drill with angled adaptor and suction irrigation, the surgeon drills away a portion of the superior and inferior vertebral bodies to provide 5 to 6 mm of vertical exposure. This is done in such a fashion that the drilling is carried more laterally as the posterior aspect of the body is approached; thus, the entire disc is not removed. Drilling is augmented by curettage as necessary to remove disc material and widen exposure. When the posterior cortical bone is reached, drilling is terminated and dissection proceeds with the angled-up curettes. Often, although not always, the posterior longitudinal ligament is opened and the dura is inspected directly. They, and subsequently Martins (9), reported satisfactory results even when multiple levels were operated. From this review, it is clear that the cervical spine seems particularly resilient to surgical efforts and, fortunately, fusion occurs in a high percentage of cases regardless of the cervical approach used. All reported results with soft lateral extruded cervical discs treated by the anterior approach with or without fusion are good. On the other hand, the results are equally good when soft lateral discs are operated posteriorly, particularly with the use of the operating microscope. The soft central extruded discs are best treated by an anterior approach.

Tew and Mayfield (23,24) have reported the complications and prevention of complications in surgery of the anterior spine. The complications of fusion include failure of fusion, anterior angulation, graft extrusion and pain, and disability from the iliac donor site. Simeone and Rothman (18) report a 3% incidence of partial graft extrusion and a 12% incidence of pseudoarthrosis with anterior fusion. Tew and Mayfield (24), reporting the results in 50 patients operated by anterior disc removal without fusion, state that fusion occurred in 100% as demonstrated by lack of motion on dynamic studies or plain radiography; bone deformity in 2%; inconsequential anterior spur formation in 8%; and adjacent spur formation in 12%. Lunsford et al. (8) report that the results of surgery in 122 cases with only anterior disc removal were no different than those in 125 cases who had anterior disc removal with fusion regardless of the type of disc herniation or the number of levels operated. Their operative complications were more frequent and hospital stay longer in fused cases. They emphasized that 66% of 253 cases with a mean follow-up of 43 months had 66% excellent or good results, 18% fair results, and 16% poor results. This differed from initial results which revealed that 77% noted immediate complete symptomatic relief. During the follow-up period, 38% noted recurrent symptoms, 51% required additional postoperative conservative care, and 38% sought further medical consultation. Four percent were reoperated at the same level, and 7% reoperated at a different level. Their report indicated that soft herniated discs had similar results to hard operated discs, but simple anterior disc removal may be preferable to anterior cervical fusion, since the results were the same, complications fewer, and hospitalization shorter without graft fusion.

It appears that simple disc removal without fusion gives results as good and perhaps better than disc removal with interbody fusion. Nerve roots and spinal cord can be adequately decompressed by simple discectomy. Osteophytes can be removed. Generally, the results are more satisfactory when soft extruded discs, either compressing a nerve root or spinal cord, are operated. This seems particularly true when only one interspace is operated. However, multiple levels have been operated with satisfactory results.

LONG-TERM RESULTS IN PATIENTS WITH SIMPLE DISCECTOMY

Using the criteria of Odom et al. (13) in which the results are graded as excellent in patients without symptoms; good in patients with mild pain that does not significantly interfere with work; fair in patients with subjective improvement but whose physical activities are limited by neck pain; and finally poor if the patient does not improve or is worse than before surgery, this author reviewed 135 patients operated between 1965 and 1979. The patients were considered in five categories: lateral extruded soft discs with nerve root compression; central soft extruded discs with spinal cord compression; chronic painful cervical discs at a single level; chronic painful discs at multiple levels; and patients with spondylotic radiculopathy and/or myelopathy. Seventy-two patients ultimately had 75 operations for lateral extruded cervical discs. Of this group, six had previous posterior partial hemilaminectomy at the same level. Four ultimately developed a soft root syndrome at an adjacent level; three were operated. Eight were readmitted for neck pain therapy during the 14-year period. Most of the ruptured discs were at the C_5 and C_6 level. I have preferred to operate the C_7 disc from the posterior approach. Excellent and good results were obtained in 85% of the cases. Fair results were obtained in 10.8% of the cases. Four patients had a definite extruded disc syndrome at an adjacent level (5.5%); one refused surgery; 95.8% of the patients benefited from the surgical procedure. Eleven percent were readmitted during the follow-up period for conservative treatment of neck pain. One patient had an extruded C_6 disc removed anteriorly and continued to complain of pain in the neck, ipsilateral, and opposite arm pain to the point where an interbody graft was required. No additional extruded fragment was found at the time of the interbody fusion. With a single disc removal, a few patients have had radicular pain and root findings in the opposite extremity as reported by Hirsch (7); however, all recovered within a month postoperative.

Eight patients presented with myelopathy due to soft cervical disc herniation. One patient had a central extrusion at an adjacent level with a recurrence of myelopathy. Three patients, including the patient with another herniation, were readmitted for therapy. Most of the central herniations occurred at C_6. None of the patients received an excellent result. However, eight received good results and one fair. None were made worse by the procedure.

The syndrome of the painful disc has been described as the patient who has mechanical pain in the neck, shoulder, and arm with or without subjective complaints of numbness or consistent neurological deficit that has been unresponsive to conservative measures for at least 6 months. Myelographic and plain X-ray changes may be present at one or more spaces, but the patient's pain and, therefore, the disc removed, were identified by the reproduction of the symptoms when a small amount of normal saline was injected into the disc. These patients frequently had X-ray evidence of one or more degenerative disc lesions. Myelographic abnormalities characterized by minor central protrusion or lateral defects were common. Thirty-three patients had a single painful disc; eleven had two painful discs. None of these cases were involved with compensation. All were considered conservative treatment failures. In an analysis of 33 single level painful discs, we noted only 51% receiving excellent and good results, with 36% receiving fair results, and poor results in 12%. Five (15%) had previous posterior partial hemilaminectomy for a soft extruded disc. Nine required readmission for conservative treatment during the period of observation. Two received excellent results, 15 good results, 12 fair results, and 4 were unimproved. It was felt that 87.5% of these patients were improved as a result of the operation. However, the percentage of excellent results is considerably less than the patients with soft extruded disc syndromes. One patient developed a profound C_6 root syndrome after anterior disc removal. At posterior operation 2 weeks later, an osteophyte was removed with pain relieved. It is recommended that, if present, osteophytes be removed because the transient anterior collapse of the interspace may narrow the foramen and produce pain and root deficit. Of the 11 patients having at least two discs removed from the anterior approach, 82% received excellent and good results; none were made worse.

Twelve operations were done on 11 patients with spondylotic radiculopathy and myelopathy. Three received excellent results, three good, three fair and three poor. Three had a previous posterior operation that failed. Three were ultimately readmitted for conservative treatment of neck pain. One had a recurrent disc at an adjacent level. Six received good and excellent results, but three were unimproved.

SUMMARY

After thorough consideration, the results from simple discectomy and discectomy with fusion indicate that fusion by bone graft is not necessary. The alarming morbidity of the anterior approach for cervical disc disease is the occurrence of another disc rupture at an adjacent level in 5.5% of our cases. Lunsford et al. (8) report 4% reoperation at the same level and 7% at an additional level. Comparing the results with the posterior partial hemilaminectomy removal of soft extruded discs as reported by Odom (13) and applying the same criteria for evaluations, results are practically identical with soft extruded discs. However, the posterior operation in the series reported by Murphey (11) from our clinic shows an incidence of a true recurrent soft fragment of 1% at the same level and 1% at an adjacent level in patients with proven initial soft lateral ruptured discs. One can only conclude that the long-term results from surgery for lateral extruded cervical discs are identical in the posterior and anterior approaches, but the anterior approach carries a greater liability of another disc at an adjacent level than the posterior approach. The chronic painful disc syndrome renders the patients improved in an incidence of approximately 87%. However, long-term good and excellent results are obtained in only 51.5% of the patients. In addition, this group frequently requires further conservative treatment for neck pain. On the other hand, in the group operated by this author, 15% of the patients had failed to get relief from neck-shoulder/arm pain with the posterior operation. It has been said that conservative treatment of patients with chronic degenerative painful disc syndromes fails to give lasting relief in 80% of the cases.

Even though I have used the saline disc injection test on a number of occasions, no conclusive significance of the test in comparing the results and the selection of the disc to be removed can be shown. The test is not recommended.

The anterior approach to the cervical spine is here to stay, but the modern neurosurgeon must be prepared to consider each surgical case individually and to determine whether the anterior or the posterior approach is preferred. With the passage of time, I have preferred to operate all but the C_7 and rare T_1 cervical discs from the anterior approach. In addition, when there is any doubt about the diagnosis, the posterior approach is preferred. If there is really a greater incidence of another extruded disc at levels adjacent to the initial disc, perhaps the indications for the routine use of the anterior approach for soft discs needs critical review. On the other hand, what is the actual incidence of disabling neck-shoulder pain in patients with extruded discs operated by posterior laminectomy? Prospective randomized comparable series of the two approaches would offer the answer to this continuing controversy.

REFERENCES

1. Bailey, R. W., and Badgley, C. E. (1960): Stabilization of the cervical disc by anterior fusion. *J. Bone J. Surg.*, 42A:565–594.
2. Boldrey, E. B. (1964): Anterior cervical decompression (without fusion). Presented at the 25th Ann. Meet. Am. Acad. Neurological Surgery, Key Biscayne, FL.
3. Cloward, R. B. (1958): The anterior approach for removal of ruptured cervical discs. *J. Neurosurg.*, 15:602–617.
4. Cloward, R. B. (1962): New method of diagnosis and treatment of cervical disc disease. *Clin. Neurosurg.*, 8:93–132.
5. DePalma, A. F., and Rothman, R. H. (1970): *The Interveterbal Discs*, pp. 154–170. W. B. Saunders, Philadelphia.
6. Hankinson, H. L., and Wilson, C. G. (1975): Use of the operating microscope in anterior cervical discectomy without fusion. *J. Neurosurg.*, 43:452–456.
7. Hirsch, D. (1960): Cervical disc rupture; diagnosis and therapy. *Acta Orthop. Scan.*, 30:172–186.

8. Lunsford, L. D., et al. (1978): The treatment of lateral cervical disc herniation by the anterior surgical approach. Presented at the Meet. Assoc. Neurological Surgeons, New Orleans, LA.

9. Martins, A. N. (1975): Anterior cervical discectomy with and without interbody bone graft. *J. Neurosurg.*, 44:290–295.

10. Mayfield, F. H. (1965): Cervical spondylosis: A comparison of the anterior and posterior approaches. *Clin. Neurosurg.*, 13:181–188.

11. Murphey, F., Simmons, J. C. H., and Brunson, B. (1972): Ruptured cervical discs, 1939 to 1972. *Clin. Neurosurg.*, 2:9–17.

12. Murphy, M. G., and Gado, M. (1972): Anterior cervical discectomy without interbody bone graft. *J. Neurosurg.*, 37:71–74.

13. Odom, G. L., Finney, W., and Woodhall, B. (1958): Cervical disk lesions. *J.A.M.A.*, 166:23–28.

14. Robertson, J. T. (1971): Anterior cervical disc removal with and without fusion. Presented at the 33rd Ann. Meet. Am. Acad. Neurological Surgery, Lake Tahoe, NV.

15. Robertson, J. T. (1972): Anterior removal of cervical discs without fusion. *Clin. Neurosurg.*, 20:259–261.

16. Robertson, J. T. (1976): Anterior operations for herniated cervical discs and for myelopathy. *Clin. Neurosurg.*, 245:250.

17. Robertson, J. T., and Johnson, S. D. (1980): Anterior cervical discectomy without fusion: Long-term results. *Clin. Neurosurg.*, 27:440–449.

18. Robinson, R. A., Walker, A. E., Ferlic, D. C., et al. (1962): The results of anterior interbody fusion of the cervical spine. *J. Bone J. Surg.*, 44A:1569–1587.

19. Simeone, F. A., and Rothman, R. H. (1975): Cervical Disc Disease. In: *Spine*, Vol. I., pp. 428. W. B. Saunders Co., Philadelphia.

20. Simmons, E. H., and Bhalla, S. K. (1969): Anterior cervical discectomy and fusion: A clinical and biomechanical study with eight-year follow-up. *J. Bone J. Surg.*, 51B:225–237.

21. Smith, G. W., and Robinson, R. A. (1955): Anterior lateral cervical disc removal and interbody fusion for cervical disc syndrome. *Bull. Johns Hopkins Hosp.*, 96:223–224.

22. Susen, A. F. (1966): Simple anterior cervical discectomy without fusion. Presented at the 27th Ann. Meet. Am. Acad. Neurological Surgery, San Francisco, CA.

23. Tew, J. M., and Mayfield, F. H. (1976): Complications of surgery of the anterior cervical spine. *Clin. Neurosurg.*, 23:424–434.

24. Tew, J. M., and Mayfield, F. H. (1979): Surgery of the anterior cervical spine: Prevention of complications. Syllabus of Hilton Head Island Neurosurgical Symposium.

Controversies in Neurology, edited by R. A. Thompson and J. R. Green. Raven Press, New York © 1983.

Surgical Treatment of Cervical Radiculopathy and/or Myelopathy: A Report Concerning 238 Operations

John R. Green, John J. Demakas*, and Apichan Pootrakul

Barrow Neurological Institute, St. Joseph's Hospital and Medical Center, Phoenix, Arizona 85013

Charles Elsberg (11), the pioneer spinal neurosurgeon, called attention to the similarity between so-called spinal chondromas and certain structures of the intact intervertebral disc as early as 1913. However, he and another generation did not trace the connection between chondromas and the intervertebral disc. An understanding of neurological syndromes, including those caused by radiculopathy and myelopathy, related to soft and hard disc protrusions, and localized and diffuse spinal stenosis has evolved slowly. From the extensive literature on these subjects, we have selected a number of contributions that have been significant in the historical and clinical development of this area of neurological surgery. These include the following publications:

1926:   Elliot (10) provided the first description of the relationship between radicular symptoms and narrowing of the intervertebral foramina in the cervical area in a case of spinal arthritis.

1927-
1928:   Schmorl's studies (43,44) elucidated the relationships of the intervertebral disc to various pathologic conditions of the vertebral column.

1928:   Stookey (53), Elsberg's successor, described clinical findings in relation to the anatomic location of ventral extradural cervical chondromas in classic fashion. Had Schmorl's studies been available, Stookey would have recognized the true nature of the lesions and would have opened up the field of intervertebral surgery earlier than 1934.

1934:   Mixter and Barr (30) are generally credited with introducing the planned surgical treatment of rupture of the intervertebral disc with involvement of the spinal canal and nerve roots. Several of their original cases involved the cervical spine.

---

*Currently Lt. Comm. (MC) USN, U.S.N.H., San Diego, California 92134

1943: Semmes and Murphey (48) accurately described the clinical findings of laterally placed cervical disc pathology, emphasized the frequency of these lesions, and predicted that most patients then being operated for supposed scalenus anticus syndrome would be found to be suffering from rupture of the cervical disc.

1944: Spurling and Scoville (51) expanded the subject of ruptured cervical intervertebral discs as a common cause of shoulder and arm pain and also the surgical techniques of cervical laminectomy, laminotomy, and the "keyhole" approach to these lesions.

1947: Kahn (23) described the role of the dentate ligaments in anterior extradural spinal masses and the mechanism of intradural and extradural decompression, including section of the dentate ligaments.

1955: Smith and Robinson (49) developed the anterior approach to the cervical spine for the treatment of cervical disc disease and myelopathy. Most of the degenerated disc was removed and a block of bone was placed in the intervertebral space under direct vision.

1956: Spurling's monograph (50) on lesions of the cervical intervertebral disc provided the modern classification of (a) soft disc protrusions, (b) hard disc protrusions, and (c) cervical spondylotic radiculopathy and myelopathy. The results of operating 197 patients in the upright position by keyhole unilateral laminotomies, partial hemilaminectomies, and by bilateral single and multiple level laminectomy, sometimes with section of the dentate ligaments, are listed.

1956: Wolf, Khilnani, and Malis (60) delineated the importance of relating the readily measurable sagittal diameter of the cervical canal to pressure changes affecting the spinal cord and nerve roots.

1958: Cloward's technique (3) of anterior cervical discectomy and fusion with a dowel of iliac bone was described and gradually became the method of choice among most neurosurgeons.

1960: Hirsch (21) first reported doing anterior cervical discectomies without fusion, with good results.

1966: Verbeist and Paz y Geuse (58) described the anterolateral approach for cervical spondylosis in cases of myelopathy or nerve root decompression.

1972: Robertson (38) reported utilization of the operating microscope, since 1965, and its advantages in anterior discectomies with and without fusion.

1978: Fager (14) discussed posterior surgical tactics for neurological syndromes of cervical disc and spondylotic lesions and recommended section of the dentate ligaments in selected patients with cervical spondylotic myelopathy, recognizing that controversy existed concerning this practice.

1979: Mayfield (29), in reporting his experiences with 800 operations for cervical spondylosis, recommended anterior discectomy with his modification of the Smith-Robinson technique for patients with spondylotic bars or discs if the spinal canals were not stenotic otherwise, and decompressive laminectomy in patients in whom circumferential myelopathy was an early manifestation and shallow stenotic canals were present. He emphasized the need for gentleness in both approaches and the advantages of the use of the air drill over customary bone instruments if bone is to be removed.

1981:   Sugar (53) reviewed in detail the pitfalls leading to spinal cord malfunction in anterior cervical discectomy, methods to avoid these complications, and techniques to treat them should they occur.

CLINICAL DATA

During a period of 42 months (January 1, 1977 to June 30, 1980), neurological surgeons of the Barrow Neurological Institute performed 238 cervical operations. Two hundred were for cervical radiculopathy, 28 for cervical myelopathy, and 10 for a combination of cervical radiculopathy and myelopathy. Anterior discectomy without fusion was the most frequent operation to be used (97 patients), laminectomy or laminotomy was next (79 patients), anterior discectomy with fusion followed numerically with 57 patients, and laminectomy with fusion was done for 5 patients. The procedures and associated clinical presentations are listed in Table 1.

The most common surgical pathology was a soft cervical disc protrusion (104 patients). Radiculopathy due to a hard disc protrusion was the next more common occurrence (80 patients). A combination of hard and soft disc protrusions was found in 22 patients. Cervical stenosis was found in 25 patients with myelopathy alone, and in 7 patients with a combination of radiculopathy and myelopathy. The clinical presentations associated with the surgical pathology, and the surgical procedures used are listed in Tables 2 and 3.

In this series of patients, males between the ages of 40 and 60 years were most commonly operated upon. Sex, age, and surgical pathology in these 238 patients are summarized in Table 4.

The most common site for soft disc, hard disc, and cervical stenosis was at the C_5 to C_6 level with C_6 to C_7 following closely in frequency of involvement. The levels, surgical pathology, and 238 operations are listed in Table 5.

TABLE 1. *Cervical operations by procedure and associated clinical presentations*

Procedure	Radiculopathy	Myelopathy	Combination	Total
Ant. discectomy	94	2	1	97
Ant. discectomy with fusion	50	4	3	57
Laminectomy	52	21	6	79
Laminectomy with fusion	4	1	0	5
Total	200	28	10	238

TABLE 2. *Surgical pathology associated with clinical presentations*

Pathology	Radiculopathy	Myelopathy	Combination	Total
Soft disc	100	2	2	104
Hard disc	80[a]	0	0	80
Soft and hard	20	1	1	22
Cervical stenosis	0	25	7	32
No. of patients	200	28	10	238

[a]One patient had two procedures.

TABLE 3. *Cervical operations: surgical pathology and surgical procedures*

	Pathology				
Operations	Soft disc	Hard disc	Soft and hard disc	Stenosis	Total
Anterior discectomy	62	25	10	0	97
with fusion	23	21	8	5	57
Cervical laminectomy	19	30	4	26	79
with fusion	0	4	0	1	5
Total	104	80	22	32	238

TABLE 4. *Surgical pathology: incidence by sex and age*

	Sex		Age		
Pathology	Males	Females	<40 yr.	40–60 yr.	>60 yr.
Soft disc	64	40	36	64	4
Hard disc	54	25	8	59	12
Soft and hard discs	14	8	1	20	1
Stenosis	22	10	3	8	21
Total	154	83	48	151	38

Previous cervical injury and previous cervical or lumbar disc surgery were occasionally factors in the medical history. These elements and the surgical pathology in this series of patients are summarized in Table 6.

Cervical Myelography

Cervical myelography with Pantopaque or Metrizamide was diagnostic and localizing in all of the 237 patients upon whom the 238 procedures were performed. As yet we have not operated for cervical radiculopathy or myelopathy on the basis of computed axial tomography alone, but we anticipate that when this technique is improved and experience warrants, CT studies of the cervical spine will be more

TABLE 5. *Levels of surgical pathology of 238 cervical operations*

Level	Soft disc	Hard disc	Soft and hard discs	Stenosis	Total
C_1–C_2	0	1	0	0	1
C_3–C_4	0	3	0	9	12
C_4–C_5	9	15	4	29	57
C_5–C_6	57	56	12	29	154
C_6–C_7	49	43	7	16	115
C_7–T_1	2	6	2	0	10
1 level	96	37	15	2	160
2 levels	8	33	7	3	51
3 levels	0	8	0	11	19
4 levels	0	2	0	7	9
5 levels	0	0	0	9	9

TABLE 6. *Medical factors[a] associated with surgical pathology*

Factors	Soft disc	Hard disc	Soft and hard discs	Stenosis	Total
Motor vehicle (16%)	17	10	1	6	39
Work injury (18%)	22	21	5	0	43
Flexion-extension (9%)	11	6	2	3	22
Anterior discectomy (2%)	1	4	0	0	5
with fusion (9%)	5	13	1	3	22
Cervical laminectomy (6%)	7	2	2	3	14
Lumbar disc symptoms (6%)	3	6	1	3	13
with surgery (13%)	9	13	5	4	31

[a]48 Additional patients lacked these factors.

TABLE 7. *Electromyography results in 100 patients*

EMG results	Myelopathy	Radiculopathy	Total
Positive	8 (62%)	34 (39%)	42
Negative	5 (38%)	53 (61%)	58
Total	13	87	100

practical. Electromyography (EMG) has been performed on 100 of our 237 patients. Table 7 summarizes the results in 13 patients with myelopathy and 87 patients with radiculopathy.

There was neither mortality nor wound infection as the result of the 238 operations for cervical radiculopathy or myelopathy.

Complications of Surgery

Transient morbidity was associated with 16 (16%) of the patients who had anterior discectomy in comparison to 15 (26%) of the patients with anterior discectomy and fusion, and 11 (13%) of the patients with laminectomy or laminotomy. These reversible complications are outlined in Table 8.

The major permanent complication, the Brown-Séquard syndrome, occurred as a result of three decompressive laminectomy procedures—all by different neurosurgical teams. Two operations were for cervical spondylotic myelopathy with marked cervical stenosis. One included three levels (C_5, C_6, and C_7) and was complicated by a postoperative epidural hematoma which was removed the same day. The patient became ambulant on the third postoperative day and was partially recovered at the time of her discharge on the twelfth postoperative day. Long-term follow-up reveals that she has made an almost complete recovery from this complication. The second procedure included five levels (C_2, C_3, C_4, C_5, and C_6), and reexploration of the spinal canal found no cause for the Brown-Séquard syndrome. The patient became ambulant on the sixth postoperative day and was partially recovered at the time of her discharge on the twenty-eighth postoperative day. Her recovery was almost complete in 1 year and she has no working disability. The third patient who suffered this complication had a three-level laminectomy and foraminotomies (C_5, C_6, and C_7) for cervical spondylotic radiculopathy. The Brown-Séquard syndrome developed over a period of three days. Myelography revealed a block at T_1 to T_2, which was found to be due to an epidural hematoma by means of T_1 laminectomy. He gradually improved, was ambulatory in 10 days, and left

TABLE 8. *Transient morbidity in 238 cervical spinal operations*

Morbidity	Anterior discectomy	Anterior discectomy with fusion	Laminectomy	Total
Donor site pain	0	12	0	12
Dysphagia	7	5	0	12
Motor deficit	3	2	6	11
Radicular pain	3	2	3	8
Cervical pain	1	2	3	6
Sensory deficit	2	1	2	5
Hoarseness	2	2	0	4
Wound hematoma	0	1	3	4
—removal	0	1	3	4
Postop. sublux.	2	0	0	2
Urinary retention	0	0	2	2
Graft extrusion	0	1 [a]	0	1
Vocal cord palsy	1	0	0	1
Pulmonary embolism	1	0	0	1
	22	29	22	73
Percentage	16%	26%	13%	18%
Patients	16	15	11	42

[a]This was a partial fusion.

the hospital on the thirty-sixth postoperative day. He persists with sufficient residual to necessitate a change of occupation.

Table 9 depicts a correlation of the number of days of hospitalization and the type of cervical spinal surgery. It is apparent that anterior cervical discectomy is associated with the shortest length of stay in the hospital, the majority of patients being well enough to be discharged on the third, fourth, and fifth days. Table 10 illustrates the number of hospital days with the surgical pathology, showing that patients who had soft discs generally went home earlier than those with other pathology.

Results of 238 cervical spinal operations have been evaluated and rated on the basis of the criteria of Odom, Finney and Woodhall (35). Their categories are:

a) *Excellent/Good*—complete or partial relief of symptoms, full activity.
b) *Fair*—improvement, some persistent limitation of activity.
c) *Poor*—no improvement, deterioration, dependent.

The clinical results of 200 operations on cervical discs (soft and hard) at the time the patients were discharged from the hospital are depicted in Table 11. Better results occurred in those patients who had anterior discectomy without fusion (88%). Long-term evaluations revealed that anterior cervical discectomy with and without fusion continued to provide relatively more excellent/good results than other procedures. However, more patients with anterior discectomy dropped from the excellent/good to the fair category as time progressed. Long-term results in operations for radiculopathy are shown in Table 12.

TABLE 9. *Postoperative hospital stay for spinal surgery*[a]

Days	Anterior discectomy	Anterior discectomy with fusion	Laminectomy	Laminectomy with fusion
1	1	0	0	0
2	5	0	0	0
3	15	2	3	0
4	22	5	6	0
5	17	4	2	0
6	12	10	8	0
7	14	15	11	2
8	1	9	10	1
9	5	5	7	0
10	1	3	9	0
11	1	1	4	0
12	0	0	4	0
13	1	0	2	0
14	0	2	1	0
>14	2	1	12	2
Patients	97	57	79	5

[a]Data is for 237 patients having 238 surgeries.

TABLE 10. *Postoperative hospital stay and surgical pathology*[a]

	Pathology				
Days	Soft disc	Hard disc	Soft and hard discs	Stenosis	Total
1	1	0	0	0	1
2	4	1	0	0	5
3	12	4	4	0	20
4	21	7	4	1	33
5	16	4	2	1	23
6	11	15	1	3	30
7	20	18	1	3	42
8	9	9	2	1	21
9	8	5	3	1	17
10	0	7	2	3	12
11	1	1	1	3	6
12	0	0	1	3	4
13	0	0	1	2	3
14	0	1	0	2	3
>14	1	7	0	9	17
	104	79	22	32	237

[a]Data is for 237 patients.

TABLE 11. *Short-term*[a] *clinical results of cervical disc operations*[b]

Procedure	Excellent/Good	Fair	Poor	Total
Anterior discectomy	83 (88%)	11 (12%)	0	94
with fusion	39 (78%)	10 (20%)	1 (2%)	50
Laminectomy	38 (73%)	11 (22%)	3 (5%)	52
with fusion	2	2	0	4
	162 (81%)	34 (17%)	4 (2%)	200

[a]Results are for 200 operations at time of discharge.
[b]Myelopathy problems excluded from data.

TABLE 12. *Long-term*[a] *clinical results of cervical disc operations*[b]

Procedure	Excellent/Good	Fair	Poor	Total
Anterior discectomy	69 (73.4%)	22 (23.6%)	3	94
with fusion	37 (74%)	10 (20%)	3	50
Laminectomy	32 (61.5%)	19 (36.5%)	1	52
with fusion	2	1	1	4
	140 (70%)	52 (26.0%)	8	200

[a]6 to 42 months after discharge from hospital.
[b]Data for 200 operations.

The clinical results of 38 operations for cervical myelopathy associated with cervical discs and cervical spondylosis and stenosis at the time of discharge from the hospital are listed in Table 13. Excellent/good results were obtained in 15 patients (40%), fair results in 20 (53%), and poor results in 3 (7%). Laminectomy was done in 28 of these operations with excellent/good results in 10 (36%), fair results in 15 (54%), and poor results in 3 (11%). Laminectomy was usually the procedure of choice for patients with cervical stenosis and anterior discectomy with or without fusion if cervical myelopathy was due to a soft or hard disc protrusion at one level. There was little significant change during an observation period of 6 to 42 months, except that two of the three patients who suffered a Brown-Séquard syndrome following decompressive cervical laminectomy improved—one to the excellent/good and the other to the fair category.

Five brief case presentations illustrate some of the clinical problems.

CASE PRESENTATIONS

Soft Disc Protrusion and Segmental Myelopathy

R. F. was a 55-year-old male who became symptom-free and returned to his usual occupation following anterior cervical discectomy and fusion at the C_6 to C_7 level (Cloward technique) in 1977. One month prior to the present admission in 1980 he noted spontaneous onset of severe neck pain with stiffness and soreness in the midcervical region associated with paresthesias of both hands and distal forearms on flexion of his neck. Examination revealed tenderness and muscle spasm in the posterior midcervical area, aggravation of paresthesias of hands on flexion of the neck with slight loss of gripping bilaterally. X-rays of the cervical spine showed a well-healed anterior cervical fusion at C_6 to C_7 level and narrowing of C_5 to C_6 and associated osteophyte changes. Cervical myelography disclosed a large anterior defect at the C_3 to C_4 level consistent with central protrusion of a soft disc fragment (Fig. 1).

Anterior microdiscectomy without the need for drilling of bone at the C_3 to C_4 level provided decompression of the spinal cord and nerve roots bilaterally and discharge from the hospital, symptom-free, on the fourth postoperative day. He returned to his usual occupation at the end of 3 weeks and remains symptom-free.

TABLE 13. *Short-term[a] clinical results for myelopathy associated surgeries*

Procedure	Excellent/Good	Fair	Poor	Total
Anterior discectomy	1	2	0	3
with fusion	4	2	0	6
Laminectomy	10	15	3	28
with fusion	0	1	0	1
Total	15 (40%)	20 (53%)	3 (7%)	38

[a]Results are for 38 operations at time of discharge from hospital.

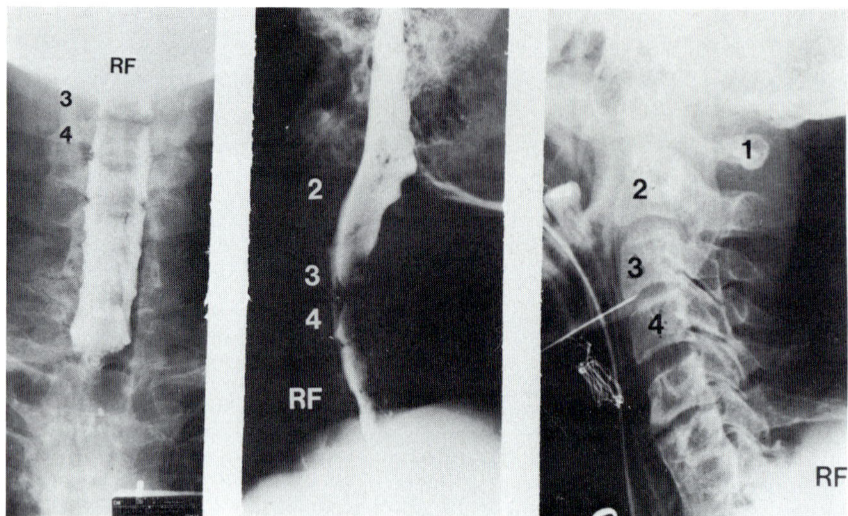

FIG. 1. Patient R. F.—Cervical myelography showing central protrusion of soft intervertebral disc, C_3 to C_4. A–P *(left)*, lateral *(middle)*, and lateral *(right)* of intraoperative film for orientation. Also shown is previous interbody fusion, C_6 to C_7, and narrowing of C_5 to C_6 disc space.

Radiculopathy and Cervical Instability Following Anterior Cervical Discectomy

R. H. was a 48-year-old male who developed cervical pain with radiation to the right shoulder and arm and associated paresthesias following an automobile accident. Anterior discectomy was done on 10/4/77 with immediate relief of his symptoms. Four days later, following an episode of strong sneezing, his cervicoradicular syndrome recurred. X-rays of the cervical spine disclosed a narrowed C_4 to C_5 disc space and posterior subluxation of C_4 to C_5 of 4 mm. Results of myelography are shown in Fig. 2. Conservative therapy failed to alleviate his discomfort, and he was referred to another neurosurgeon.

Operation on 12/22/77 consisted of removing disc material and osteophytic spurs bilaterally and fusion with a dowel of iliac bone (Cloward technique) at the C_4 to C_5 level. He was discharged from the hospital on the seventh postoperative day in an improved condition but was readmitted 8 days later because of recurrence of his symptoms. The C_4 to C_5 dowel of bone was found to project anteriorly for 5 mm and the mild preoperative subluxation of C_4 to C_5 was still present. He improved with conservative care over a period of 5 days in the hospital and recovered excellently over a period of the next 3 months. When reevaluated 1 year later, he had become disabled because of lumbar disc problems, but he was satisfied with the results of his cervical surgery. X-rays showed excellent fusion and alignment of his cervical spine. This patient represents a complication of anterior discectomy that was corrected by further anterior discectomy and fusion.

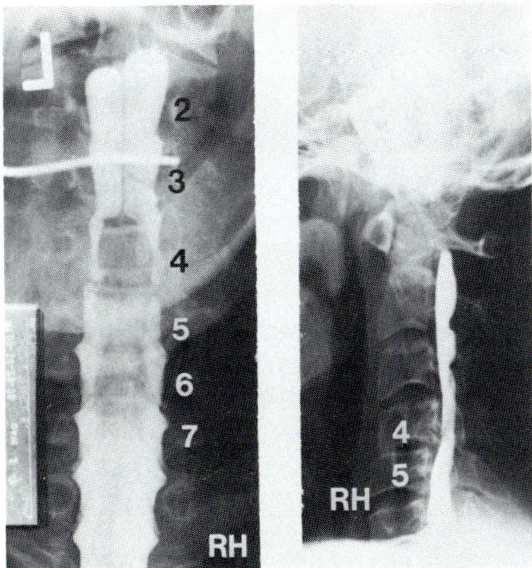

FIG. 2. Patient R. H.—Cervical myelography showing extradural compression at C_4 to C_5 *(right)* and minimal ventral protrusion with narrowed disc C_4 to C_5.

Cervical Spondylosis and Radiculopathy

G. D. was a 48-year-old male who developed cervical pain with radiation to the left shoulder and arm with intermittent numbness of the second, third, and fourth digits of the left hand over a period of 4 months. He also complained of interscapular pain on the left side. Head turning to the left would trigger pain. Examination disclosed a decreased range of motion of his neck, tenderness over the spinous process of C_6, and a decreased left triceps reflex. There were no convincing motor or sensory changes.

X-rays of the cervical spine showed cervical spondylotic changes in the C_5 to C_7 regions with narrowing of the C_6 to C_7 interspace. Electromyography demonstrated early changes suggestive of left C_7 radiculopathy. Cervical myelography disclosed spondylotic-stenotic defects of C_4 to C_7, maximally at C_6 to C_7 (Fig. 3). Operation consisted of anterior microdiscectomy and removal of osteophytes bilaterally aided by Hall microair drill and curettes at the C_6 to C_7 level. The patient was not relieved of radicular pain at the time of his discharge from the hospital on the eighth postoperative day.

He was readmitted 4 days later because of increasing pain. Decreased biceps and brachioradialis reflexes were elicited on the left, and decreased sensation in the distribution of the seventh cervical dermatome was found on the right side. Electromyography showed persistence of the C_7 radiculopathy on the left and neurogenic weakness in the same segments on the right. An orthopedic consultant recommended decompression from the posterior approach, fusion, and a halo brace. A psychiatric consultant found him to be depressed. A halo brace was applied 2 weeks following admission. Cervical laminectomy of C_5 to C_6 and foraminotomies at C_5 to C_6 and

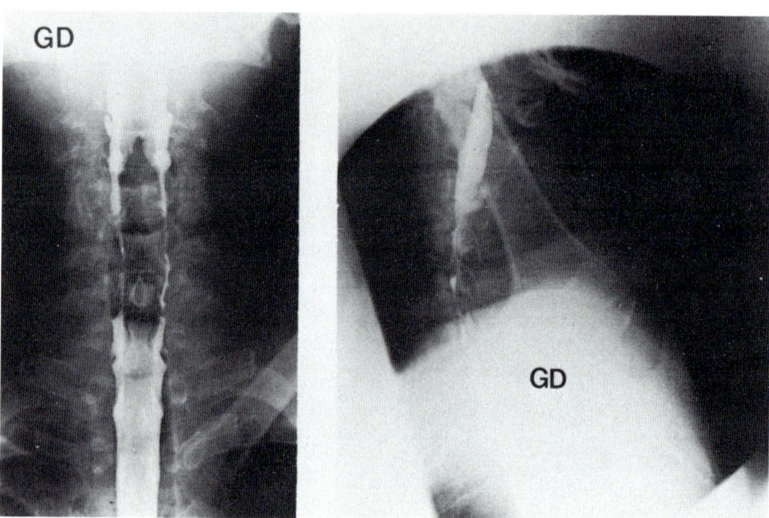

FIG. 3. Patient G. D.—Cervical myelography showing cervical spondylosis with stenosis at C_4 to C_7, A–P and lateral views, maximally at C_6 to C_7.

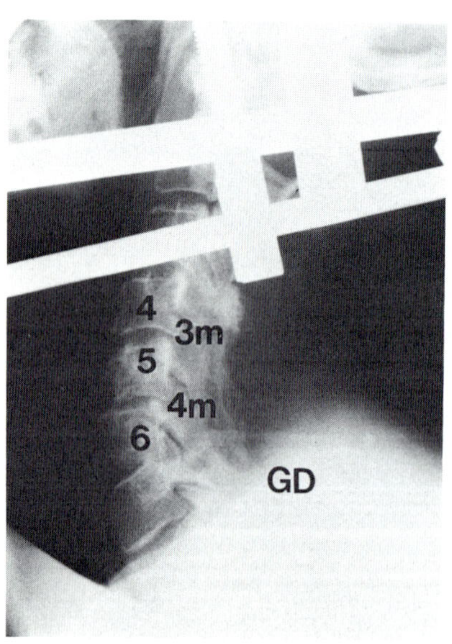

FIG. 4. Patient G. D.—Lateral C-spine with patient in halo following posterior fusion of C_4 to C_7, showing subluxation posteriorly of C_4 on C_5 of 3 mm and of C_5 and C_6 of 4 mm.

C_6 to C_7 were done bilaterally, followed by fusion of C_4 to C_7 in the halo brace (Fig. 4). The arm pain subsided gradually, bilateral triceps weakness was marked, and his emotional problems worsened. The triceps and intrinsic hand muscles remained weak. He received inpatient rehabilitation and psychiatric care for 2 months. Follow-up X-rays showed some minor subluxation at C_5 to C_6 and EMG studies disclosed denervation potentials of C_5 through T_1 bilaterally, particularly on the right side.

Retrospectively, in view of the clinical syndrome and the myelographic abnormalities, decompressive laminectomy, foraminotomies and fusion of C_4 to C_7 should have been the operation of choice initially.

Radiculopathy Due to Soft Disc Extrusions at Two Levels

S. R. was a 49-year-old male who felt a catch in his left interscapular region as he pulled on a wrench on 9/9/79. Pain in this area persisted associated with pain across the left shoulder to the lateral arm area. He was obliged to stop working 2 days after the injury and noted the gradual development of weakness and atrophy of the proximal musculature of the left shoulder. X-rays of the cervical spine showed minimal degenerative disc changes at the C_5 to C_6 level. Electromyography demonstrated evidence of C_5 nerve root involvement on the left side. Cervical myelography showed an anterior extradural filling defect at C_4 to C_5 and C_5 to C_6 with a lateral filling defect at C_4 to C_5 on the left as well as widening of the root sleeve at C_5 to C_6 on the left (Fig. 5). The C_4 to C_5 defect was more impressive than the C_5 to C_6 defect and it was decided that an anterior cervical discectomy at the C_4 to C_5 level was indicated, but that if insufficient pathology was found to account for the syndrome at the C_4 to C_5 level, a similar procedure at the C_5 to C_6 level would be performed. Operation on 12/5/79 consisted of anterior cervical discectomy

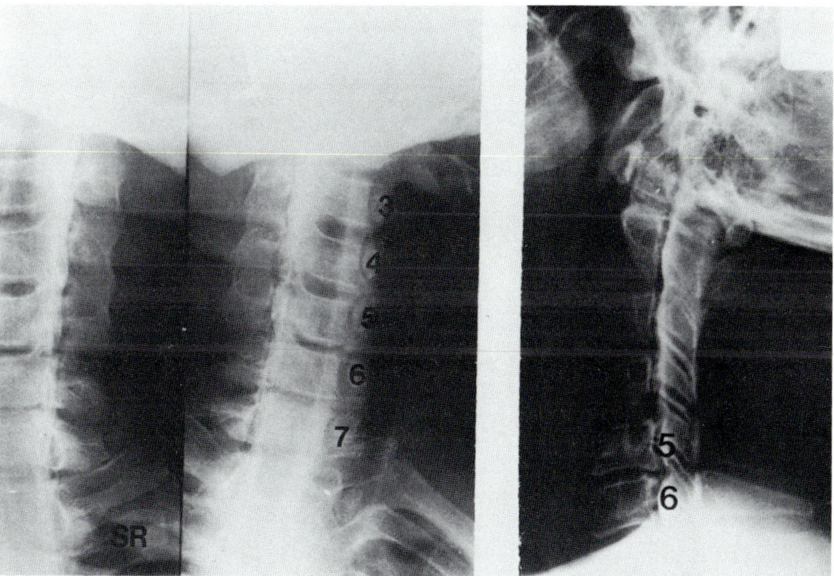

FIG. 5. Patient S. R.—Oblique views of cervical myelography showing root sleeve defects of C_4 to C_5 and to a lesser extent C_5 to C_6. Lateral view shows protruded soft discs with C_5 to C_6 being more prominent than C_4 to C_5.

at the C_4 to C_5 level. Extruded disc fragments in the extradural space on the left side were removed. Magnification loupes (4.5 powered) and a headlight were used. This articulation was found to be unstable. The patient improved significantly but did not become pain free. He returned to work, but because of progressive disability due to persistent problems, he was readmitted by the same neurosurgeon.

Myelography showed a ventral bar with partial obstruction and focal cord widening at the C_5 to C_6 level (Fig. 6). Because of the significant C_5 to C_6 myelography changes and persistent radicular pain, anterior discectomy at C_5 to C_6 was advised. Operation consisted of C_5 to C_6 anterior discectomy with excision of a soft disc protrusion and removal by curettage of osteophyte formations encroaching upon the intervertebral foramina and posterior origins of the vertebral bodies. At the time of the last reevaluation he was planning to return to his prior occupation as a mechanic.

Cervical Spondylotic Myelopathy

J. C. is a 69-year-old internist who had experienced stiffness and soreness of his neck over a period of 20 years. In 1974, he noted numbness of the thumb, index,

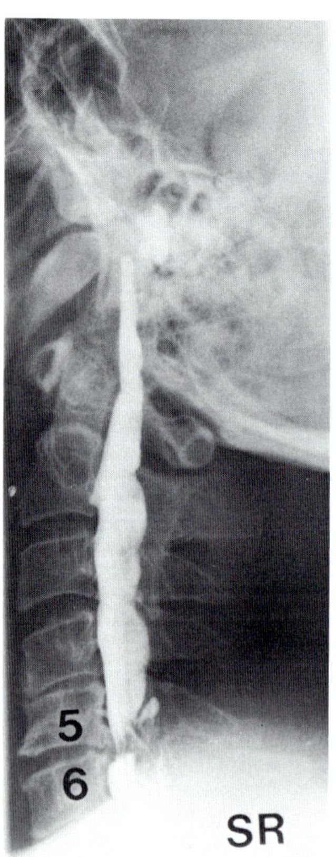

FIG. 6. Patient S. R.—Lateral cervical myelogram illustrating postoperative narrowing of C_4 to C_5 disc without evidence of ventral myelographic defect and localized stenotic lesion at C_5 to C_6 primarily due to spondylitic ridge ("hard disc protrusion").

and middle fingers. Gait disturbance; falling due to periodic weakness of the legs; loss of skilled movement in both hands (worse on the left); numbness of the thumb, index, and middle fingers of both hands; and stiffness and soreness of the neck became progressively more disabling over a 6-month period prior to admission. Nocturia and slowness of urinary flow were attributed to prostatism. Examination revealed a marked gait disturbance with unsteadiness, uncertainty, lurching, and broadness of base. Neck motion was restricted. Finger-to-nose testing was normal but gross dysmetria was evident on heel-to-knee examination bilaterally. Motor power was preserved except for the flexors of the thumbs and index fingers. The thenar eminences were shiny and wrinkled bilaterally. The deep reflexes were 4 + in the upper extremities and 2 + in the lower extremities. Hoffmann and Babinski reflexes were absent. Vibratory sensation was absent in the right lower extremity and decreased in other extremities. Hypalgesia was limited to the radial aspects of the hands and adjacent distal forearms. X-rays of the cervical spine showed advanced cervical spondylosis and stenosis.

Myelography demonstrated severe ridging and stenosis at C_3 to C_4 and lesser involvement at C_4 to C_5 in the anterior-posterior views and marked stenotic spondylotic changes of the lower half of C_3, all of C_4, and a portion of C_5 on lateral views (Fig. 7). Operation consisted of decompressive laminectomy of C_3, C_4, and C_5. Upon opening the dura, it was observed that the spinal cord was located

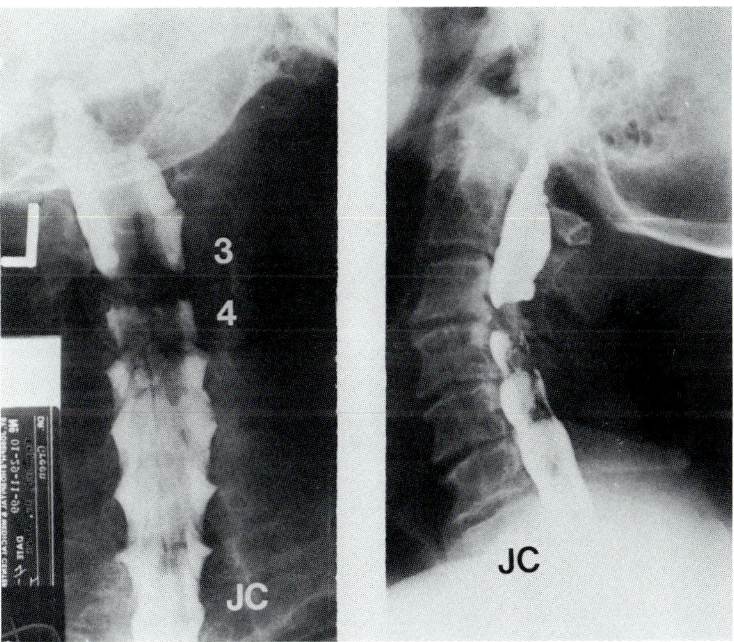

FIG. 7. Patient J. C.—Cervical myelography. A–P view *(right)* showing severe ridging and stenosis at C_3 to C_4 and lesser involvement at C_4 to C_5. Lateral study *(left)* depicts marked stenotic spondylitic lesion of lower half of C_3, all of C_4, and a portion of C_5.

anteriorly and that following section of the dentate ligaments at C_3 and C_4 bilaterally the cord was seen to float posteriorly. The patient's postoperative recovery was gratifying with rapid recovery from pain, weakness, numbness, gait disturbance, and sphincteric dysfunction. Within a period of three months, he resumed his practice, and at the end of 6 months reported that his recovery was complete.

There may be controversy about the tethering effects of dentate ligaments but this type of experience is impressive.

DISCUSSION

Modern cervical disc surgery was introduced by Semmes and Murphey (48), Spurling and Scoville (51), and Brain et al. (2) following earlier pioneering contributions (11,36,52). Spurling's monograph (50) in 1956 provided an excellent summation of the status of posterior cervical decompressive surgery, at the beginning of the anterior cervical fusion era.

The introduction by Smith and Robinson (49) in 1955 of the anterior approach to the cervical spine for the treatment of cervical disc disease and myelopathy was remarkably accelerated by Cloward (3) in 1958 with his technical advances, instrumentation, methodology, and follow-up reports (4–6) regarding removal of discs and osteophytes, anterior interbody fusion, complications, and results. Cloward also observed that immobilization by anterior cervical fusion could reduce the spurring existent in the fixed segments. Scoville (45) pointed out, in 1961, that when several vertebrae are fixed by cervical spondylosis or by anterior cervical fusion, that there was an increased susceptibility for the discs above and below to herniate or to degenerate and cause spur formations.

The first anterior discectomy without fusion was reported by Hirsch (21) in 1960 with improvement in 70% of his patients, with no evidence of instability and with spontaneous fusion in some patients. He pointed out that distressing pain on the opposite side occurred occasionally in the postoperative period. This approach was supported in 1964 by Boldrey (1) and subsequently by Susen (54), Murphy and Gado (32), Robertson (38–40), Martins (27), Hankinson and Wilson (20), Dunsker (9) Lunsford et al. (25,26), and Guarnaschelli and Dzenitis (18), among others. The trend to manage cervical discs whether they are of the soft or hard categories by the anterior approach is illustrated in our 200 operations. The majority were operated by eight neurosurgeons or by their senior neurosurgical residents. Ninety-four procedures (47%) were anterior cervical discectomies without fusion, and 50 operations (25%) were anterior cervical discectomies with fusion. Thus the anterior approach was selected for 144 of the 200 operations for cervical discs, or in 72% of the operations.

Shortly after the introduction of microsurgery, the operating microscope was adapted to anterior cervical discectomy procedures with and without fusion, by Robertson, in 1965, and first reported by him in 1972 (38). Hankinson and Wilson (20) discussed anterior cervical microdiscectomies without fusion in 52 patients with equally satisfactory results when the procedures were done at single or multiple levels. The use of the operating microscope for cervical disc surgery has been amplified by Martins (27), Hoff and Wilson (22), Robertson (39–40), and Williams (59). In the present series, 30 of the 144 anterior approaches were microsurgical. We observe a trend to use the microscope more than operating loupes among the neurosurgeons on our staff. It is apparent to the authors that the microscope, with the assistance of the vertebral spreader, allows excellent visualization and exposure of the dura and nerve roots in patients with soft and hard discs, including those in which the disc space is significantly narrowed. It is rarely necessary to use a drill under these circumstances. Although promising, anterior microdiscectomy has not been proven to provide more excellent/good long-term results in the surgical treatment of cervical discs than other procedures, as yet.

Cervical myelopathy is the most serious consequence of cervical disc herniation and cervical spondylosis, and it may also be associated with a wide variety of congenitallesions that can diminish the caliber of the cervical spinal canal. Developmental cervical stenosis implies an inborn narrowing of the sagittal diameter of the canal. Mechanical factors may create intraspinal encroachment and cervical myelopathy, and can be immediate, as with fractures and fracture dislocations, or chronic, as with rheumatoid arthritis, Paget's disease, inflammatory and granulomatous lesions, metabolic diseases, and with calcification and ossification of the posterior longitudinal ligament.

The importance of the sagittal diameter of the bony cervical spinal canal and its significance in cervical spondylotic myelopathy and radiculopathy were pointed out by Wolf et al. (60). Of equal importance in planning these surgical procedures is the recognition of lateral spinal canal constrictions and foraminal alterations (12). Myelography, with either Pantopaque or Metrizamide, is an essential study to determine the extent of cervical stenosis. A sagittal diameter of 10 mm or less and widening of the spinal cord greater than 17 mm in the C_4 to C_7 levels are diagnostic of cervical stenosis and possible cervical myelopathy (12). Crandall et al. (8,17) have identified five clinical syndromes in cervical spondylotic myelopathy. These syndromes are: (a) the transverse lesion, (b) the motor system, (c) the mixed brachialgia and cord, (d) the Brown-Séquard, and (e) the central cord syndrome. From the era of Elsberg (11) until Smith and Robinson (49) introduced anterior cervical disc removal and fusion to treat cervical radiculopathy and myelopathy, the procedure of choice for these conditions was the posterior approach by means of laminectomy. In 1934, the same year that Mixter and Barr (30) established intervertebral disc protrusion as a cause of radiculopathy, Peet and Echols (36) successfully removed a cervical disc causing myelopathy by laminectomy. Currently, cervical spondylotic myelopathy, associated with cervical stenosis or by more localized soft or hard discs, is being treated entirely from the posterior approach (14), from the anterior approach (8,20,22), or with the procedure being selected according to the clinicoradiological data (13,28,38). Nine of the 38 patients with cervical myelopathy in our series were treated by anterior cervical procedures. The surgical pathology in these instances was soft disc protrusions at one level or hard disc protrusions associated with cervical spondylosis at one or two levels. Decompressive laminectomy was utilized if there was cervical stenosis in three or more levels or if there was also significant narrowing of the canal posteriorly or laterally. Mayfield's experience (29) with 800 operations for cervical spondylosis included 21 instances of cervical myelopathy due to acute central herniation of a disc fragment and 41 patients with spondylotic cervical myelopathy. His recommendations for selecting the appropriate operation are:

a) For acute myelopathy—excision of the herniated disc fragment by either route, depending upon the surgeon's experience. He prefers his modification of the anterior Smith-Robinson technique.

b) For chronic myelopathy—the anterior approach if the spinal canal is not stenotic, and the posterior approach if the cervical canal is stenotic, shallow, and when circumferential myelopathy is an early clinical manifestation.

The mortality rate for operations to treat cervical radiculopathy and myelopathy is extremely low. Murphey et al. (31) had no deaths in 648 operations for ruptured cervical discs, all but 25 being done by the posterior approach. They preferred the prone position because of the possibility of air embolism. A single death in an anterior decompressive procedure for cervical spondylotic myelopathy was reported by Lunsford et al. (26)—a mortality rate of 3% for 37 similar operations, but 0% mortality in 253 anterior surgeries for cervical discs. Our series reports no mortalities in 238 procedures, 38 being for cervical myelopathy.

Wound infection rates are frequently not included in publications of results, but have been reported from 0 to 3% [0% our series, and (25); 1% (56,58); 1.6% (25); 2% (22); and 3% (26)].

The length of hospital stay following various cervical spinal procedures reflects that the least transient morbidity is with anterior discectomy, the next least with anterior cervical fusion, and the most with laminectomy (see Table 9). Robinson, Walker and Ferlic (42) reported an incidence of complications of 18%, and Connolly et al. (7) reported complication in 51% of the patients after anterior discectomy and fusion. Robertson (38) commented that complications of anterior cervical spinal surgery appeared to be greater than with posterior hemilaminectomy, particularly if the prone position was used, and that the incidence of additional soft disc rupture in an additional space was 2 to 3% with the anterior approach in comparison to 1% with the posterior approach. Some settling of the vertebrae occurs if fusion is not done, anteriorly more than posteriorly, but spontaneous fusion occurs, usually in 3 months.

Hoff and Wilson (22), Schmidek (42), and Tew and Mayfield (55,56) have reported similar complications of surgery of the anterior cervical spine, including:
1. Injuries to the soft tissue related to the surgical exposure
    (a) Perforation of the pharynx, esophagus, and/or trachea
    (b) Vocal cord paresis due to injury of the recurrent laryngeal or vagus nerve
    (c) Vertebral artery injury
    (d) Pneumothorax
    (e) Cerebrospinal fluid fistula
    (f) Horner's syndrome

(g) Carotid artery or jugular vein injury
(h) Postoperative hematoma
(i) Wound infections
2. Spinal cord or nerve root injuries
3. Problems related to bone fusion
    (a) Failure of fusion
    (b) Angulation deformity
    (c) Aseptic necrosis and discitis
    (d) Extrusion of bone graft
    (e) Infection, seroma, hematoma
    (f) Painful hip

Hoff and Wilson (22) reported an incidence of 3% retractor related injury; a 2% incidence of wound infection, osteomyelitis, and discitis; nonunion with or without interbody grafting in 10%; transient postoperative neck and interscapular pain in 20% of patients with resolution in a few weeks; and worsening of the neurological deficit in 5% of the patients treated by microsurgical approach to the anterior cervical spine and spinal cord. Lunsford et al. (25) reported that the most troublesome operative complication in 253 anterior cervical operations for disc herniation was vocal cord paresis—seven instances of the fused hard disc cases with two being permanent. The next most bothersome complication involved extrusion of the bone graft in six patients, three requiring reoperation. There was a 23% incidence of complications after anterior cervical discectomy and fusion. Transient morbidity in our series (Table 8) was 16% for anterior discectomy alone; 26% for anterior cervical discectomy and fusion; and 13% for laminectomy, hemilaminectomy, or "key-hole" laminotomy procedures—an overall incidence of transient morbidity of 18%. Analysis of six patients who developed myelopathy following anterior cervical discectomy and fusion by six different neurosurgeons who were defendants in professional liability litigation, and suggestions regarding prevention and treatment, by Sugar (53), is recommended reading for neurosurgeons, orthopedists, and their residents.

The results of surgery for cervical radiculopathy and cervical myelopathy by means of anterior, posterior, and occasionally both procedures have been well documented, but much controversy continues regarding optimal measures due to multifactorial variables in the selection process.

Spurling (50) reported the results of medical and surgical treatment of 197 patients with rupture of the cervical disc in 1956. His 61 operations were done in the sitting position and consisted of: (a) the "key-hole" unilateral approach, (b) hemilaminectomy, and (c) laminectomy. He reported 90% improvement. However, if the method of ranking of results of Odom et al. (35) is applied, 61.3% would be in the excellent/good category. Murphey et al. (31) reported that similar surgery from 1939 to 1969 had returned 319 of 350 patients to their presurgical occupations. This represents 90% excellent/good results. These neurosurgeons objected to the upright position because of the possibility of air embolism and operated their patients in the prone position. However, their entire series of operations involved 648 patients in 33 years. A follow-up of 380 patients was possible from 1 to 28 years and 350 patients responded regarding their working status. These data point up the difficulties in comparing statistical results of surgical procedures.

Our results for cervical disc surgery from the posterior approach are excellent/good in 61.5% of the patients in the long-term and more closely resemble those of Spurling (61.3%).

Recent reports of operations for cervical discs from the posterior approach (14,46,47) provide data with which to compare the results of other procedures. Scoville (46) reports good to excellent results in 95% of their patients with lateral cervical discs and in 64% of his patients with central bar ridge discs. Guarnaschelli and Dzenitis (18) obtained excellent/good results in 83% of 75 patients with posterior cervical discectomy.

The results of operations for cervical discs from anterior approaches are also somewhat difficult to evaluate because of variable analytic data, i.e., the use of the word "improved" to include excellent/good and fair results, contrary to the rankings recommended by Odom et al. (35). Hirsch (21) reported 70% "improvement" with anterior discectomy without fusion, Hoff and Wilson (22) indicated that 90% of their patients undergoing anterior cervical microdiscectomy were relieved of their symptoms, if a bony spur of disc fragment was removed, and 70% obtained significant improvement in cases of cervical spondylotic radiculopathy by similar operations. Robertson (40) described 85% excellent and good results following anterior microdiscectomy for soft discs, fair results in 10.8%, with overall "improvement" in 95.8% of the patients. In operations for the "painful disc syndrome" the early results were excellent/good in 87.5% of the patients, but dropped to 51.5% with long-term follow-up. Lunsford et al. (25) found excellent/good results with 72% of the patients with soft discs, with 65% of the patients with hard discs following anterior cervical microdiscectomy, and indicated that 88% were "improved" based upon the sum of 69% excellent/good and 19% fair results. They found somewhat similar results following anterior cervical discectomy and fusion operations (66% excellent/good plus 15% fair results—or 81% improved). Guarnaschelli et al. (18) tallied 96% excellent/good results following anterior cervical microdiscectomy for cervical discs and 92% excellent/good results after anterior cervical discectomy and fusion. Our results are tabulated in Table 11 (short-term) and Table 12 (long-term) and show somewhat similar results to those published by other neurosurgeons and suggest little long-term differences between patients operated with and without fusion for cervical discs.

All reports indicate that the short- and long-term results of spinal surgery for cervical myelopathy are less satisfactory than for radiculopathy whether the cause is a disc protrusion, soft or hard, or stenosis associated with a number of causes, including cervical spondylosis (8,15,17,19,26,34,37,40,57). The best results appear to be associated with the excision of a soft disc from either the posterior or anterior approach. Robertson (40) has reported excellent/good results in 8 of 8 patients (100%) following anterior cervical microdiscectomy for soft discs, and 50% for cervical spondylotic myelopathy. Hoff and Wilson (22) reported 40% excellent/good results for anterior microdiscectomy, Gregorious et al. (17) 50%, Lunsford et al.

(26) 50% (20% excellent/good and 30% fair results) after discectomy, and 60% (24% excellent/good and 26% fair results) after discectomy and fusion. Guarnaschelli et al. (18) reported similar results. Our results are tabulated in Tables 13 and 14 regarding 38 operations for cervical myelopathy. The natural history and prognosis, including spinal cord impairment, of cervical spondylosis have been well described by Lees et al. (24) and Nurick (33,34). Beneficial long-term effects on the process of cervical myelopathy have been reported by means of anterior discectomy (17) and by laminectomy (16,36,46). It is apparent that each patient requires detailed study and individual consideration in order to make the decision whether surgical intervention is warranted.

SUMMARY

The primary goal in the surgical treatment of cervical radiculopathy and/or myelopathy is to decompress the involved structures by removing the offending "soft" or "hard" disc fragment or osteophyte or other causes of cervical stenosis at single or multiple levels.

In caring for these conditions, neurological surgeons have five surgical options when conservative means of therapy have failed in patient rehabilitation. These options are anterior cervical discectomy (ACD); anterior cervical discectomy with fusion (ACD + F); posterior cervical decompression (PCD) by means of "key-hole" laminotomy and foraminotomy, hemilaminectomy and laminectomy at one or more levels; posterior cervical decompression with fusion (PCD + F); and Verbeist's anterolateral operations. In that the clinical syndromes and conditions are widely variable, there are indications for multiple types of surgical therapy.

The adaption of microneurosurgery to cervical procedures, particularly with the anterior approach, has increased the precision and simplicity of these operations. As yet, there is no incontestable evidence that microdiscectomy has significantly improved the percentage of long-term results. However, the authors have adopted this tactic for some time and plan to analyze comparable series of patients in the future.

Anterior cervical microdiscectomy with or without fusion and posterior cervical decompressive procedures have similar outcomes on the long-term basis. However,

TABLE 14. *Long-term[a] clinical results of operations for cervical myelopathy*

Procedure	Excellent/Good	Fair	Poor	Total
Anterior discectomy	1 (33.3%)	2 (66.7%)	0	3
with fusion	1 (16.7%)	5 (83.3%)	0	6
Laminectomy	12 (42.8%)	15 (53.5%)	1	28
with fusion	0	1	0	1
	14 (36.8%)	23 (60.5%)	1	38

[a]Results are for 38 operations 6–42 months after discharge from hospital.

there is an increased morbidity with fusion procedures. A slight but definite deterioration in the operative results with long-term follow-up studies was most apparent with laminectomy for spondylotic myelopathy (20%), followed by anterior cervical discectomy (19%), posterior cervical decompressive procedures (12%), and least for anterior discectomy with fusion (6%) in our series of 238 operations. The reduced morbidity associated with anterior cervical microdiscectomy and significant reduction of days of hospitalization are cogent reasons why this procedure is preferable in most instances, except in patients with cervical instability, in multiple level cervical stenosis, in C_7 to T1 discs, or if there is a question about the diagnosis, i.e., a possible intraspinal neoplasm. Whereas cervical spondylosis with or without myelopathy can be treated very satisfactorily at single or multiple levels by means of anterior cervical microdiscectomy, decompressive laminectomy is preferred if there is measurable decrease in the sagittal diameter ($<$10 mm) over three or more levels. Under these conditions, the dentate ligaments are sectioned if the cord is found to be tethered to the anterior structures by these ligaments.

A prospective randomized study of ACD, ACD + F, PCD, and PCD + F procedures for the treatment of cervical radiculopathy and myelopathy is needed to answer the many questions about the selection of procedures for these conditions. Meanwhile, the optimal operation for each patient must be individualized, based upon all available information, and the training and experience of the neurosurgeon.

ACKNOWLEDGMENT

The authors wish to express appreciation for the invaluable assistance provided by Georgia Frederic in the preparation of this manuscript.

REFERENCES

1. Boldrey, E. B. (1964): Anterior cervical decompression (without fusion). Presented at the *25th Ann. Meet. Acad. Neurological Surgery*, Key Biscayne, FL.
2. Brain, W. R., Knight, G. D., and Bull, J. W. D. (1948): Discussion on rupture of the intervertebral disc in the cervical region. *Proc. R. Soc. Med.*, 41:509–516.
3. Cloward, R. B. (1958): The anterior approach for removal of ruptured cervical discs. *J. Neurosurg.*, 15:602–617.
4. Cloward, R. B. (1962): New method of diagnosis and treatment of cervical disc disease. *Clin. Neurosurg.*, 8:93–132.
5. Cloward, R. B. (1963): Lesions of the intervertebral discs and their treatment by interbody fusion methods: The painful disc. *Clin. Orthop.*, 27:51–57.
6. Cloward, R. B. (1974): *Ruptured cervical intervertebral discs. Removal of disc and osteophytes and anterior interbody fusion.* Signature Series 4. Codman and Shurtleff.
7. Connolly, E. S., Seymour, K. J., and Adams, J. E. (1965): Clinical evaluation of anterior cervical fusion for degenerative disc disease. *J. Neurosurg.*, 23:431–437.
8. Crandall, P. H., and Batzdorf, U. (1966): Cervical spondylotic myelopathy. *J. Neurosurg.*, 25:57–66.
9. Dunsker, S. B. (1981): Cervical spondylotic myelopathy: Pathogenesis and pathophysiology. In: *Cervical Spondylosis*, edited by S. B. Dunsker, pp. 119–134. Raven Press, New York.
10. Elliot, G. R. (1926): A contribution to spinal arthritis involving the cervical region. *J. Bone J. Surg.*, 8:42–52.
11. Elsberg, C. A. (1913): Experiences in spinal surgery: Observations upon 60 laminectomies in spinal disease. *Surg. Gynec. Obstet.*, 16:117–132.

12. Epstein, B. S., Epstein, J. A., and Jones, M. D. (1978): Anatomoradiological correlations in cervical spine disease and stenosis. *Clin. Neurosurg.*, 25:148–173.
13. Epstein, J. A., Carras, R., Lavine, L. S., and Epstein, B. S. (1969): The importance of removing osteophytes as part of the surgical treatment of myeloradiculopathy in cervical spondylosis. *J. Neurosurg.*, 30:219–226.
14. Fager, C. A. (1978): Posterior surgical tactics for the neurological syndromes of cervical disc and spondylitic lesions. *Clin. Neurosurg.*, 25:218–244.
15. Galera, G. R., and Tovi, D. (1968): Anterior disc excision with interbody fusion in cervical spondylotic myelopathy and rhizopathy. *J. Neurosurg.*, 28:305–310.
16. Gorter, K. (1976): Influence of laminectomy on the course of cervical myelopathy. *Acta Neurochir.*, 33:265–281.
17. Gregorious, F. K., Estrin, T., and Crandall, P. H. (1976): Cervical spondylotic radiculopathy and myelopathy. A long-term follow-up study. *Arch. Neurol.*, 33:618–625.
18. Guarnaschelli, M. D., and Dzenitis, A. J. (1982): Anterior cervical discectomy without fusion: Comparison study and follow-up. *(In preparation)*.
19. Guidetti, B., and Fortuna, A. (1969): Long-term results of surgical treatment of myelopathy due to cervical spondylosis. *J. Neurosurg.*, 30:714–721.
20. Hankinson, H. L., and Wilson, C. B. (1975): Use of the operating microscope in anterior cervical discectomy without fusion. *J. Neurosurg.*, 43:452–456.
21. Hirsch, D. (1960): Cervical disc rupture: diagnosis and therapy. *Acta Orthop. Scandin.*, 30:172–186.
22. Hoff, J. T., and Wilson, C. B. (1978): Microsurgical approach to the anterior cervical spine and spinal cord. *Clin. Neurosurg.*, 26:513–528.
23. Kahn, E. A. (1947): The role of the dentate ligaments in spinal cord compression. *J. Neurosurg.*, 4:191–199.
24. Lees, F., and Turner, J. W. A. (1963): Natural history and prognosis of cervical spondylosis. *Br. Med. J.*, 2:1607–1610.
25. Lunsford, L. D., Bissonette, P. A.-C., Janetta, P. J., Sheptak, P. E., and Zorub, D. S. (1980a): Anterior surgery for cervical disc disease. Part 1: Treatment of lateral cervical disc herniation in 253 cases. *J. Neurosurg.*, 53:1–11.
26. Lunsford, L. D., Bissonette, P. A.-C., Janetta, P. J., Sheptak, P. E., and Zorub, D. S. (1980b): Anterior cervical surgery for cervical disc disease. Part 2: Treatment of cervical spondylotic myelopathy in 32 cases. *J. Neurosurg.*, 53:12–19.
27. Martins, A. N. (1975): Anterior cervical discectomy with and without interbody bone graft. *J. Neurosurg.*, 44:290–295.
28. Mayfield, F. H. (1966): Cervical spondylosis: A comparison of anterior and posterior approaches. *Clin. Neurosurg.*, 13:181–188.
29. Mayfield, F. H. (1979): Cervical spondylotic radiculopathy and myelopathy. In: *Advances in Neurology*, Vol. 22, edited by R. A. Thompson and J. R. Green, pp. 307–321. Raven Press, New York.
30. Mixter, W. J., and Barr, J. S. (1934): Rupture of the intervertebral disc with involvement of the spinal canal. *N. Engl. J. Med.*, 211:210–215.
31. Murphey, F., Simmons, J. C. H., and Brunson, B. (1973): Ruptured cervical discs, 1939 to 1972. *Clin. Neurosurg.*, 20:9–17.
32. Murphy, M. G., and Gado, M. (1902): Anterior cervical discectomy without interbody fusion. *J. Neurosurg.*, 37:71–74.
33. Nurick, S. (1972a): The pathogenesis of the spinal cord disorder associated with cervical spondylosis. *Brain*, 95:87–100.
34. Nurick, S. (1972b): The natural history and the results of surgical treatment of the spinal cord disorder associated with cervical spondylosis. *Brain*, 95:101–108.
35. Odom, G. L., Finney, W., and Woodhall, B. (1958): Cervical disc lesions. *J.A.M.A.*, 166:23–28.
36. Peet, M. M., and Echols, D. H. (1934): Herniation of the nucleus pulposus. A cause of compression of the spinal cord. *Arch. Neurol. Psychiatry*, 32:924–932.
37. Phillips, D. G. (1973): Surgical treatment of myelopathy with cervical spondylosis. *J. Neurol. Neurosurg. Psychiatry*, 36:879–884.
38. Robertson, J. T. (1972): Anterior removal of cervical disc without fusion. *Clin. Neurosurg.*, 20:259–261.

39. Robertson, J. T. (1981): Anterior cervical discectomy without fusion. In: *Cervical Spondylosis*, edited by S. B. Dunsker, pp. 181–190. Raven Press, New York.

40. Robertson, J. T. (1982): This volume.

41. Robinson, R. A., Walker, A. E., Ferlic, D. C., and Wiecking, D. K. (1962): The results of anterior interbody fusion of the cervical spine. *J. Bone J. Surg. (Am.)*, 44:1569–1587.

42. Schmidek, H. H. (1977): The anterolateral approach to the cervical spine in the management of cervical spondylosis and its complications. In: *Current Techniques in Operative Neurosurgery*, edited by H. Schmidek and W. Sweet, pp. 303–322. Grune and Stratton, New York.

43. Schmorl, G. (1927): Die pathologische Anatomie die Wirbelsäule. *Ver. d. Deutsch. Orthop. Gesselbsch.*, 21:3–40.

44. Schmorl, G. (1928): Zur Kenntis der Wirbelkorperepiphyse und der an ihr vorkommenden Verletzungen. *Arch. f. klin. Chir.*, 153:35–45.

45. Scoville, W. B. (1961): Cervical spondylosis treated by bilateral facetectomy and laminectomy. *J. Neurosurg.*, 18:423–428.

46. Scoville, W. B. (1981): Cervical disc: Classification, indications, and approaches with special reference to posterior keyhole operation. In: *Cervical Spondylosis*, edited by S. B. Dunsker, pp. 155–166. Raven Press, New York.

47. Scoville, W. B., Dohrmann, G. J., and Corkill, G. (1976): Late results of cervical disc surgery. *J. Neurosurg.*, 45:203–210.

48. Semmes, R. E., and Murphey, F. (1943): Syndrome of the unilateral rupture of the sixth cervical intervertebral disc, with compression of the seventh cervical nerve root. *J.A.M.A.*, 121:1209–1214.

49. Smith, G. W., and Robinson, R. A. (1955): Anterior lateral disc removal and interbody fusion for cervical disc syndrome. *Bull. Johns Hopkins Hosp.*, 96:223–224.

50. Spurling, R. G. (1956): *Lesions of the Cervical Intervertebral Disc*. American Lecture Series. Charles C Thomas, Springfield, Illinois.

51. Spurling, R. G., and Scoville, W. B. (1944): Lateral ruptured cervical intervertebral discs: A common cause of shoulder and arm pain. *Surg. Gynecol. Obstet.*, 78:350–358.

52. Stookey, B. (1928): Compression of the spinal cord due to ventral extradural cervical chondromas. *Arch. Neurol. Psychiatry*, 20:275–291.

53. Sugar, O. (1981): Spinal cord malfunction after anterior cervical diskectomy. *Surg. Neurol.*, 15:4–8.

54. Susen, A. F. (1966): Simple anterior cervical discectomy without fusion. Presented at the *27th Ann. Meet. Am. Acad. Neurological Surgery*, San Francisco, CA.

55. Tew, J. M., Jr., and Mayfield, F. H. (1976): Complications of surgery of the anterior cervical spine. *Clin. Neurosurg.*, 23:424–434.

56. Tew, J. M., Jr., and Mayfield, F. H. (1981): Surgery of the anterior cervical spine: Prevention of complications. In: *Cervical Spondylosis*, edited by S. B. Dunsker, pp. 191–208. Raven Press, New York.

57. Verbeist, H. (1973): The management of cervical spondylosis. *Clin. Neurosurg.*, 20:262–294.

58. Verbeist, H., and Paz y Geuse, H. D. (1966): Anterolateral surgery for cervical spondylosis in cases of myelopathy or nerve root decompression. *J. Neurosurg.*, 25:611–622.

59. Williams, R. W.: Microcervical foraminotomy: A surgical alternative for intractable radicular pain. *(In preparation)*.

60. Wolf, B. S., Khilnani, M., and Malis, L. I. (1956): The sagittal diameter of the bony cervical spinal canal and its significance in cervical spondylosis. *J. Mt. Sinai Hosp.*, 23:283–292.

Controversies in Neurology, edited by R. A.
Thompson and J. R. Green. Raven Press,
New York © 1983.

Medical Versus Surgical Treatment of Metastatic Spinal Cord Tumors

William R. Shapiro and Jerome B. Posner

*Memorial Sloan-Kettering Cancer Center, Department of Neurology,
New York, New York 10021*

At Memorial Sloan-Kettering Cancer Center (MSKCC) we see 60 to 80 patients with epidural spinal cord or cauda equina compression each year. Most of these patients have far advanced systemic cancer, but occasionally spinal cord compression is the presenting complaint. In all patients, if the disorder is not effectively treated, it will progress to paraplegia or quadriplegia which, once established, is irreversible. If the diagnosis can be made early, and the patient treated vigorously, paralysis can often be avoided or reversed. Because the signs frequently develop rapidly, spinal cord compression must be considered an emergency, requiring immediate diagnosis and treatment.

The purpose of this review is to consider the forms of treatment available in this disorder. "Medical" treatment consists of corticosteroid hormones administered immediately on diagnosis, and megavoltage radiation therapy (RT). "Surgical" treatment consists of decompression of the spinal cord or cauda equina with removal of as much tumor as possible followed by medical treatment as defined above. Thus, we are not addressing the question of surgical therapy as such versus medical therapy, but whether surgery *adds* to the effectiveness of medical therapy. In the discussion that follows, epidural spinal cord compression is defined as tumor directly compressing the spinal cord or tumor compressing the cauda equina. Since the results of therapy do not differ in the two sites, they can be lumped together.

An important issue when considering the value of surgical and medical therapy is how one evaluates the results. Improvement in pain is important, as are changes in motor and sphincter function, but the most important component is ambulation. Ambulation is easily assessed, has a specific endpoint, and can be followed over time. A change in sensory level is less important functionally than whether or not the patient can walk. In our series from MSKCC, ambulation has been the major variable assessed, but pain and sphincter function are also important, and are also evaluated.

THE SYNDROME

Epidural spinal cord compression comes about because tumor invades and narrows the epidural space, directly compressing the cord, the venous structures in the epidural space, or the feeding radicular arteries; the latter producing secondary vascular changes in the cord. The commonest site of the initial metastasis is the vertebral body and pedicles, especially with cancer from breast, lung, or prostate. Lymphomas tend to arise in the paravertebral regions and produce spinal cord compression by infiltration through the intervertebral foramina. A small number of patients have epidural spinal cord metastasis by hematogenous routes. Intramedullary metastases occur in only about 4% of patients. In our series from MSKCC, the commonest tumor producing epidural spinal cord compression was breast cancer in women, followed by lung cancer primarily in men, prostate cancer, and then the genitourinary tumors (6,7). Lymphomas accounted for a large number of epidural spinal cord compressions in the old series (6) but are seen less frequently as therapeutic modalities for the primary lesion have improved.

The first symptom in almost all patients with epidural spinal cord compression is pain. The pain usually, but not always, precedes motor or sensory symptoms. The median duration of such pain prior to the onset of weakness in our own series was approximately 7 weeks, and ranged from 1 day to 2 years. In the cervical and lumbar regions, the pain tends to be radicular plus local, while in the thoracic region, the pain is more commonly local without a radicular component. Weakness occurs in three-fourths of patients who present with epidural spinal cord compression, and bladder and/or bowel dysfunction occurs in nearly 60%. The degree of weakness varies. Approximately one-half of our patients are still able to ambulate when they are seen, while a little over one-third are paraparetic and bedridden. Fortunately, the incidence of paraplegia has fallen *peri passu* with the increased awareness of this complication among physicians taking care of patients with cancer. Approximately 15% of our patients are paraplegic at the time of presentation. Sensory loss occurs in three-fourths of patients, and deep tendon reflex abnormalities occur in about 65%. Myelography performed by lumbar puncture usually indicates a complete or near complete spinal cord block. At MSKCC we routinely place radio-opaque contrast material above the block, either by cisternal puncture or by lateral C_{1-2} puncture, to define its upper limit. Once a diagnosis is established by myelography, patients are given large doses of corticosteroid hormones, usually dexamethasone 100 mg intravenously immediately, and then the decision is made about further therapy. One interesting result of our more recent study (7) is that the steroids may themselves account for much of the pain relief that occurs from treatment.

CLINICAL STUDIES

The results of therapy of epidural spinal cord compression at MSKCC have been reported in detail by Gilbert et al. (6) and in a later series by Greenberg et al. (7). In the Gilbert series, 235 patients were reviewed retrospectively; in the later series, an additional 83 patients were reported who received a modified radiation schedule. In the former series, patients were assigned to receive RT alone or surgery plus

RT purely on the basis of the clinical judgment of the neurologist or neurosurgeon seeing the patient. This study was not controlled, and the patients were not randomized. Patients with lymphoma usually received RT. Patients who were paraplegic at the time they were initially seen usually received RT alone. Surgical decompression was carried out in order to establish a definitive diagnosis in the event that the nature of the primary tumor had not previously been established. RT in the Gilbert et al. (6) series consisted of 400 rads daily for 3 days to the local port, followed by 200 rads daily to a total of 2,000 to 4,000 rads. In the later series (7), a specific RT trial was attempted in which patients received 500 rads per day for each of 3 days, followed by a 4 day rest, and then 300 rads a day for 5 additional days. In the initial series, patients were treated with dexamethasone at 16 mg daily in divided doses, whereas in the later series patients received the initial high dose of 100 mg of dexamethasone with tapering over the next 12 days.

The results in the Gilbert et al. (6) series were as follows: Of 170 patients treated with RT alone, 84 ambulated (49%), and of 65 patients treated with a combination of RT plus surgery, 30 ambulated (46%). This difference was not statistically significant. Generally, patients who were ambulatory before therapy did best; of the Grade I (or ambulatory) patients, 79% of those who received RT walked after treatment, and 64% of those who had surgery plus RT walked. Grade II patients (those who were paraparetic) were helped equally by RT alone or surgery plus RT; 45% in each series walked post-treatment. Paraplegic patients did poorly; only 1 of 29 patients walked after RT, and 1 of 10 patients walked after surgery plus RT. So-called radiation-sensitive tumors, i.e., seminoma, lymphoma, myeloma, Ewing's sarcoma, and neuroblastoma, were treated equally effectively by RT alone and by surgery plus RT. More impressively, the so-called less radiation-sensitive tumors, i.e., carcinoma, melanoma, and soft tissue sarcoma, also fared about equally well between RT and RT plus surgery. Of 131 patients given RT alone, 59 (45%) walked, and of 50 patients treated with surgery plus RT, 19 (38%) ambulated afterwards. Because rapid progression of spinal cord dysfunction has traditionally represented an indication for surgery, an analysis was performed on the results of 22 patients whose weakness developed over 48 hours. Of 9 patients who underwent surgical decompression, none improved, while of 13 patients receiving RT without surgery, 7 improved, a difference which statistically favored the group receiving RT alone. The long-term results depended as much on the nature of the tumor, and therefore how well the patients did systemically, as it did on the initial form of treatment. For example, of 12 surgically treated patients who maintained or regained ambulation, 9 remained ambulatory for 6 months or longer. Of 47 patients successfully treated by RT alone, 78% of those alive after 6 months remained ambulatory. Generally, however, patients with myeloma, lymphoma, and breast cancer did better than those with lung cancer or cancer of the genitourinary tract. In this retrospective series, surgery appeared to add little to RT as a primary treatment mode. Patients generally did poorly, with only about half of the patients ambulating after therapy. The addition of surgery did not substantially improve this result. Nevertheless, the results strongly indicated that when patients were treated early they did much better, and when patients entered the hospital walking, they had a 75% chance or better of leaving the hospital walking.

In the Greenberg et al. (7) series, all 83 patients received RT alone. Of patients who were Grade I (ambulatory), 34 of 38 patients (89%) ambulated after treatment. Of paraparetic patients who could move their legs against gravity (Grade II), 42% ambulated after treatment; whereas of 13 patients who were not able to move their legs against gravity (Grade III), 3 (23%) ambulated, and none of 8 patients who were paraplegic (Grade IV) ambulated. The new RT protocol as described above did not appear to be any more effective than the prior, more prolonged form of RT. One interesting finding in this series was that in association with high-dose steroid therapy, patients had rapid and complete amelioration of pain with minimal morbidity. Once again, breast cancer patients fared best with 52% ambulating, whereas lung cancer patients did less well, with only 27% ambulating.

Surgical series of some interest include that of Livingston and Perrin (10), who reviewed 100 patients treated with surgical decompression. Surgical decompression produced effective pain relief in 70% of the patients, and 58 of 100 patients could walk postoperatively, including 5 of 20 patients who had been paraplegic. Of these 5, 2 had cauda equina compression. Not clear in the report was the extent of RT utilized in these patients; apparently many had been radiated prior to the surgical decompression, but several also received RT after surgery. Cobb et al. (3) reported a retrospective series of patients with breast cancer treated for epidural spinal cord compression: 26 patients underwent initial laminectomy followed by RT, and 18 received RT alone. Of 9 patients who were able to walk, 7 retained that ability after laminectomy and RT, an identical figure to 7 of 9 patients who received initial RT alone. Of patients who could not walk, 6 of 17 treated by initial laminectomy walked (35%), and 5 of 9 treated with RT only (56%) walked. These investigators concluded that there was no advantage to initial surgery over that afforded by RT alone. Pain improved in 46% of the patients receiving initial laminectomy, and in 72% of patients treated by RT alone. Dunn et al. (5) reviewed their 15-year experience of combined decompressive laminectomy and radiation therapy in treating 104 patients with metastatic epidural spinal compression. Despite the fact that both ambulation and the less precise "improvement in motor strength" were used to evaluate the results, only 33% of patients improved and 23% were worse. A more recent series was that reported by Young et al. (13), who attempted a prospective study of RT alone versus surgery plus RT. Twenty-nine patients were randomly assigned to undergo a laminectomy followed by RT or RT alone. (The RT schedules were not quite the same in the two groups—the postoperative RT consisted of 3,000 rads given in 10 divided doses over 14 days, while RT alone consisted of 400 rads per day for 3 days, and 1,800 rads administered in 7 equally divided doses over 14 days.) Of 6 patients who were initially ambulatory and treated with surgery plus RT, 3 (50%) continued to walk, and all 5 of 5 patients who were initially ambulatory and treated with RT alone walked. Of 9 nonambulatory patients treated with surgery plus RT, 4 walked (44%), while 2 of 6 nonambulatory patients treated with RT alone walked (33%). Of 3 patients who were paraplegic, 1 treated with surgery plus RT failed to improve, and 2 treated with RT alone also failed to improve. There was similarly little difference in the results at 4 months, with an approximately equal response in both groups. Improved sphincter function and pain relief were produced approximately equally with both forms of treatment. Of interest was the fact that patients who had a complete block on myelography did less well than patients who had only a partial block. Unfortunately, the degree of block was not equally distributed among the two groups: more patients in the surgery plus RT group had a complete block than did patients in the RT alone group. Surgery in this series consisted of posterior laminectomy.

Other series describing surgical excision of spinal metastases have been reviewed by Black (1). All are retrospective, and Black concludes that on the average, RT by itself is superior to surgery by itself and there is no difference between RT plus surgery versus RT alone.

Complications of treatment are important in evaluating the effectiveness of therapy. Black (1) in his review found on average a 9% death rate in the first month after surgical decompression. In part, this high figure reflects death due to cancer but not related to the surgery. Indeed, mortality has fallen considerably over the last 20 years with the improvement of surgical techniques, but morbidity remains high. Surgical complications include wound infection, wound dehiscence, epidural hematoma, cerebrospinal fluid fistula, meningitis, and spinal instability. Even in the series of Livingston and Perrin, 10% of their patients had significant morbidity (10). Morbidity following RT alone is less easily defined, although there is always some concern about late radiation myelopathy. In patients with short-term survival, this appears to be an inconsequential concern.

One other point about surgery needs to be made which concerns the value of surgical fusion techniques for spinal instability. It is generally thought that RT per se will not improve the instability of a spine badly damaged by tumor. Various fusion techniques have been recommended in this circumstance (4,8). It should be pointed out, however, that necrotic tumor is soft, and that the relatively severe kyphotic deformities that are occasionally seen in such patients produce less neurological deficit than would be expected from a similar deformity in nontumorous bone. Not infrequently, we see patients who have severe angulation, especially of the cervical spine, who can be treated effectively with simple cervical collars and RT, and who do not require fusion techniques. Nevertheless, this is a point which has not been adequately studied.

LESSONS FROM THE LABORATORY

While our experience with epidural spinal cord compression at MSKCC is extensive, we realized several years ago that there were basic questions about such spinal cord compression which could not be answered in the patient. For example, we could not determine directly what the pathogenesis of the spinal cord compression was, i.e., was it specifically direct spinal cord compression or did it relate as well to vascular damage? Did epidural spinal cord compression produce edema in the underlying spinal cord, and could steroids treat such edema? At what point was paraplegia irreversible and, of course, what was the best mode of therapy? With these questions in mind, we developed a model of epidural spinal cord compression using the Walker 256 carcinoma in the rat (12). Subsequently, Ikeda et al. (9) developed a similar model in the rabbit using VX_2 tumor. The results of the laboratory studies so far have led to changes in the clinical methods of handling these patients and have produced some initial answers to the questions posed above. The studies by Ushio et al. (12) clearly demonstrated the presence of edema in underlying spinal cord compression. Edema also occurred in the rabbit model of epidural spinal cord compression by tumor (9). This edema appeared to be vasogenic, and was proportional to the degree of weakness (12). In the rat model it was effectively treated by dexamethasone in relatively high dosages (12). It was the high dosage of the steroids that led us to attempt similar high-dose steroid therapy in our patients, and led to the 100 mg dexamethasone dose sequence. Epidural tumor impinged early on the epidural venous plexus and the resultant stasis may have contributed to edema (9). Later the tumor compressed arteries and reduced the blood flow to the cord, although infarction was always a late complication (12). In subsequent studies (11), we showed that a number of treatment modalities were effective. Dexamethasone clearly improved the animals but the effect was transient. A five vertebral laminectomy centering over the area of spinal cord compression and performed under a dissecting microscope produced only minimal improvement, with the animals rapidly becoming paraplegic. The most effective therapy in the Walker 256 tumor model was cyclophosphamide, but the tumor itself is highly sensitive to that form of treatment, and therefore these results were less applicable to patient care. RT was effective, however, and in a number of different experiments we showed that high initial RT dosage followed by continued RT was the most effective means of treatment and was better than single doses, lower doses alone, or continuous low-dose treatment. These results permitted us to attempt the RT schedule reported by Greenberg et al. (7). One of the more important results of the animal studies was that paraplegic animals could be effectively treated. Cyclophosphamide cured the animals even after they had become paraplegic, and the best RT schedule also permitted animals to ambulate. These data suggested that if a patient has only recently become paraplegic, aggressive treatment should be undertaken because of the potentiality for improvement.

DISCUSSION

In reviewing the clinical series, it is clear that there is little "controversy" in the problem of managing epidural spinal cord compression. There is no evidence that surgery adds to the effectiveness of RT in the treatment of these patients. If a patient is still walking at the time he develops spinal cord block, he has a very good chance of maintaining his ability to walk whether treated by RT alone or by surgery plus RT. If he is paraparetic, however, the chances are only about 50/50 that he will ever walk again. If a patient is paraplegic, he has little chance of walking again. Furthermore, surgery is not without complications. A 10% morbidity is an important consideration in a patient paraparetic from epidural spinal compression. One must consider the risk of converting a patient who may become paraplegic because his tumor does not respond to RT into a patient who may be similarly paraplegic but also have a wound dehiscence and require additional nursing care for this complication. Furthermore, the majority of surgical procedures done on such patients are posterior procedures, laminectomies, done to "decompress" the spinal cord. Since 85% of carcinomas affect the vertebral bodies, the laminectomy frequently increases the instability of the spine since it removes the remaining supporting elements.

One important consideration in the issue of surgery is why operations do *not* help. It is a tenet of neurosurgery that a laminectomy decompresses the spinal cord by permitting it to ride out of the compressed area. This tenet may not be correct, however, since in most patients the tumor lies anterior in the vertebral body and the compression force is from anterior to posterior. Removing the posterior elements does indeed permit the spinal cord to spring backwards, but what is not clear is how this maneuver, which does not itself relieve the pressure produced from the anterior tumor, allows neurological function to be restored. There is also the claim that this is the only method of assuring an open spinal canal. Our experience at MSKCC indicates that up to 30% of spinal canals are still blocked postoperatively. We have already alluded to the problem of instability created by operating on the posterior elements when the vertebral body is destroyed. This is another reason for the failure of surgery to improve patients. Surgery also may potentially compromise the vessels, especially the radicular feeding arteries, and that may hasten infarction. Perhaps the most important reason that surgery fails is that to relieve compression on a spinal canal, one must remove the compressing mass. Since most of this mass lies anteriorly, posterior laminectomy fails to accomplish this goal.

How then might surgery help? Conceptually, one needs to go where the tumor is and, hence, an anterior approach, especially in the neck, or an anterolateral approach in the thorax would appear to be a more rational choice than a laminectomy. The procedure of an anterior decompression, popularized by Cloward (2) and commented on by a number of investigators (1,4,8), permits removal of the tumor contained in the vertebral body and therefore permits removal of the compressing spinal cord mass. Such a procedure also spares the posterior components, which are usually normal, and therefore does not further compromise the stability of the spinal column. The procedure also permits spinal fusion, either by bone grafts (4) or by acrylic inserts (8). It would seem that if operations are to *add* to the treatment of this disease, the procedures of choice would appear to be anterior tumor excision with or without spinal fusion. There is evidence that such techniques frequently permit patients, especially those with unstable spines, to return to a more normal life (4). Further investigational work along these lines would seem to be indicated.

The question must also be raised of whether there is a need for a prospective study comparing RT alone with RT plus initial surgery. We do not believe that such a study is indicated. Despite its retrospective nature, the available evidence is overwhelming that surgery does not contribute to the effectiveness of RT in the treatment of epidural spinal cord compression. The recent small prospective study by Young et al. (13) is consistent with this conclusion. Considering the reasons for failure of posterior decompression, we see no reason to perform such a study in the large group of patients that would be needed to demonstrate even moderate differences. Rather, we would encourage neurosurgeons to improve anterior or anterolateral techniques and, having done this, then consider such a prospective study.

For the present we recognize two indications for surgery: the absence of a histologic diagnosis of tumor, and recurrent symptoms in a patient previously radiated to the same site. Although we occasionally operate on patients who continue to progress despite RT, we recognize that the chances of success in such circumstances are low (6). There may continue to be some indication for surgery in patients with readily accessible tumor or tumor that is highly radioresistant, although here too, greater success than that achieved with RT alone is not to be expected.

Finally, it would seem prudent to continue the effort to improve methods of therapy of cancer per se. Our animal studies indicate that when a tumor is sensitive, as is Walker 256 to cyclophosphamide, we could cure the animal's paraparesis as well as the tumor by effectively treating the tumor itself. This similarly appears to be the case for epidural spinal cord compression from lymphoma. Our studies indicate that the best results, regardless of the mode of therapy, occur in relatively sensitive tumors like breast cancer. Thus, even in dealing with the neurological complications of systemic cancer, we face the same problems as does the oncologist. The treatment of the complications of cancer consists of the treatment of the cancer itself, and only as that treatment improves will the treatment of the complications improve.

REFERENCES

1. Black, P. (1979): Spinal metastasis: Current status and recommended guidelines for management. *Neurosurgery*, 5:726–746.
2. Cloward, R. B. (1962): New method of diagnosis and treatment of cervical disc disease. *Clin. Neurosurg.*, 8:93–132.
3. Cobb, C. A., Leavens, M. E., and Eckles, N. (1977): Indications for nonoperative treatment of spinal cord compression due to breast cancer. *J. Neurosurg.*, 47:653–658.
4. Conley, F. K., Britt, R. H., Hanbery, J. W., and Silverberg, G. D. (1979): Anterior fibular strut graft in neoplastic disease of the cervical spine. *J. Neurosurg.*, 51:677–684.
5. Dunn, R. C., Kelly, W. A., Wohns, R. N. W., and Howe, J. F. (1980): Spinal epidural neoplasia. *J. Neurosurg.*, 52:47–51.
6. Gilbert, R. W., Kim, J.-H., and Posner, J. B. (1978): Epidural spinal cord compression from metastatic tumor: Diagnosis and treatment. *Ann. Neurol.*, 3:40–51.
7. Greenberg, H. S., Kim, J.-H., and Posner, J. B. (1979): Epidural spinal cord compression from metastic tumor: Results with a new treatment protocol. *Ann. Neurol.*, 8:361–366.
8. Hansebout, R. R., and Blomquist, G. A. (1980): Acrylic spinal fusion: A 20-year clinical series and technical note. *J. Neurosurg.*, 53:606–612.
9. Ikeda, H., Ushio, Y., Hayakawa, T., and Mogami, H. (1980): Edema and circulatory disturbance in the spinal cord compressed by epidural neoplasms in rabbits. *J. Neurosurg.*, 52:203–209.
10. Livingston, K. E., and Perrin, R. G. (1978): The neurosurgical management of spinal metastases causing cord and cauda equina compression. *J. Neurosurg.*, 49:839–843.

11. Ushio, Y., Posner, R., Kim, J-H., Shapiro, W. R., and Posner, J. B. (1977): Treatment of experimental spinal cord compression caused by extradural neoplasms. *J. Neurosurg.*, 47:380–390.
12. Ushio, Y., Posner, R., Posner, J. B., and Shapiro, W. R. (1977): Experimental spinal cord compression by epidural neoplasms. *Neurology*, 27:422–429.
13. Young, R. F., Post, E. M., and King, G. A. (1980): Treatment of spinal epidural metastases. *J. Neurosurg.*, 53:741–748.

Controversies in Neurology, edited by R. A. Thompson and J. R. Green. Raven Press, New York © 1983.

Surgery, Radiation, and Chemotherapy in the Treatment of Malignant Brain Tumors

Philip H. Gutin and Victor A. Levin

Brain Tumor Research Center and the Departments of Neurological Surgery and Radiation Oncology, School of Medicine, University of California, San Francisco, California 94143

Complete surgical resection of a malignant brain tumor is seldom possible, and the search for highly effective antitumor agents has been unproductive. Although the growth of malignant brain tumors can be slowed, their cure remains one of the greatest challenges to clinical oncology.

Since extra-axial tumors that derive blood supply primarily or entirely from the meningeal, cranial, and scalp vessels present different surgical, biological, and pharmacological problems from parenchymal tumors, we confine this discussion of therapy for malignant brain tumors to the primary and metastatic parenchymal tumors.

SURGERY

With the aid of computerized tomography (CT), we can diagnose brain tumors earlier than in previous decades. Unfortunately, a tumor has usually grown at least 2 cm in diameter before clinical signs and symptoms appear and before the diagnosis is confirmed by a CT scan. Anaplastic astrocytomas are often larger than 4 cm in diameter by the time radiation therapy is initiated (32), at which point the tumor contains in excess of 10^{10} cells (greater than 30 g) and a significant population of nonproliferating (G_0) cells.

The surgical cure of any tumor is limited primarily by metastasis and local invasion. Since primary brain tumors seldom metastasize, metastasis complicates their resection less frequently than it does the resection of tumors elsewhere in the body. Local invasion, however, is a barrier to adequate surgical resection in virtually every case. Extensive resection of malignant brain tumors is also difficult because of the network of thin-walled blood vessels that enter, exit, and course within them. These vessels, especially those associated with high-flow arteriovenous shunts, bleed freely, and the usual hemostatic maneuvers are frequently ineffective in closing transected neoplastic arteries in the brain.

The goal of good cancer surgery is to aggressively resect the maximum amount of neoplasm. When total resection is not possible, cytoreductive surgery contributes measurably to the efficacy of subsequent chemotherapy in many solid tumors; presumably, the success of the adjuvant therapy is directly related to the increased fractional cell kill (per unit drug dose) that is possible in smaller tumors. The impressive results of adjuvant chemotherapy and/or irradiation in patients with breast carcinoma and osteogenic sarcoma are directly related to the extensive resection that can be accomplished in these areas.

A malignant brain tumor cannot be cured by surgery alone; extensive surgical resection is precluded by the tumor's invasion of cerebral areas that subserve critical neurological functions. Even the most aggressive resection of a malignant glioma can achieve little more than a 1 log reduction in the tumor cell population, leaving more than 10^9 cells to be eradicated by radiation and chemotherapy. Under these circumstances, the subsequent therapy can hardly be considered adjuvant to surgery. Given the surgical accessibility of most malignant brain tumors, and the probability of a better response to chemotherapy after the reduction of tumor burden, the only rational approach is to resect the tumor as extensively as possible. A decision to forego surgery, or to perform only a needle biopsy, subverts the patient's interest in all but the most extreme cases.

For the success of brain tumor therapy to equal that achieved in other areas, it would be necessary to reduce the residual tumor cell population to a point where it no longer exceeds the cell kill potential of available oncolytic agents. In view of the invasive character of malignant gliomas, this may be an unlikely prospect.

RADIATION

Radiation therapy is the modality that has proved the most effective against malignant brain tumors. Results from the Brain Tumor Study Group (BTSG) showed that patients with primary malignant brain tumors who received more than 5,000 rads to the whole brain survived 20.5 weeks longer than patients treated by surgery alone (58). Analyzing these data critically, Walker et al. found there were stepwise increments in survival in patient cohorts receiving 5,000, 5,500, or 6,000 rads (62). Higher doses of photon radiation than these, however, expose the patient to a significant risk of brain necrosis (49). Because necrosis of normal brain precludes the administration of more than 6,000 to 7,000 rads at the conventional dose-rates, there is a search for ways to improve the therapeutic ratio. We have focused on two methods: (a) increasing the sensitivity of hypoxic tumor cells to conventional radiation doses, and (b) increasing the radiation dose to the tumor while sparing adjacent normal brain by interstitial implantation of the radiation source.

Hypoxic Cell Radiosensitizers

Oxygen effect

Although it may seem likely that hypoxic tumor cells would be more vulnerable to radiation than the oxygenated cells, Holthusen (27) reported, as early as 1921, that in the absence of oxygen, *Ascaris* eggs were radioresistant. Thirty years later,

Gray et al. investigated the radiobiology of the oxygen effect and its importance in the radiation therapy of solid tumors (20). Studying histological sections of bronchial carcinomas with reference to areas of necrosis and their distance from blood vessels, Thomlinson and Gray observed that viable tumor cells were never found more than 180 μm from a blood vessel (54). They speculated that tumor cells could not flourish without adequate oxygen or nutrients from the circulating blood. Independent of this histological observation, they calculated that oxygen would diffuse through tissue only to a distance of 150 to 200 μm from a capillary, at which point the oxygen tension would be zero. From the close correlation between these observed and calculated values, they concluded that oxygen was the critical nutrient in maintaining tumor cell viability.

Between the oxygenated cells clustered close to capillaries and the anoxic, necrotic cells 150 to 200 μm from capillaries, there is a zone of cells with low oxygen tension (Fig. 1). It is thought that the radioresistance of these borderline hypoxic cells is represented in the terminal tail with an abruptly decreased slope that is seen on radiation survival curves obtained for most experimental solid tumors.

Figure 2 illustrates the impact of the oxygen effect on radiation cell kill. For cultured mammalian cells irradiated in an environment of nitrogen (hypoxia), the dosage required to produce any specified reduction in subsequent cell survival is three times greater than that required for cells irradiated in an oxygen environment;

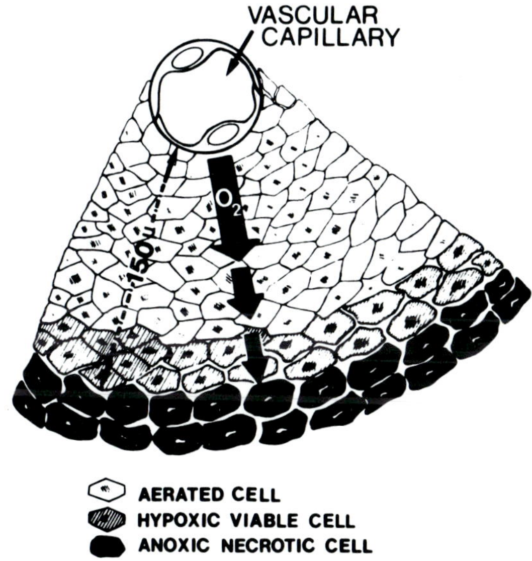

FIG. 1. Oxygen diffusion from a capillary is limited by uptake from respiring tumor cells. Between the oxygenated cells close to the capillary and the necrotic cells 150 to 200 μm away, there is a zone of cells with oxygen tension high enough for the cells to be viable, but too low for them to be radiosensitive. These hypoxic cells may be a barrier to cure by irradiation. (Reproduced with permission from E. J. Hall, *Radiobiology for the Radiologist*, 2nd ed., Harper & Row, 1978.)

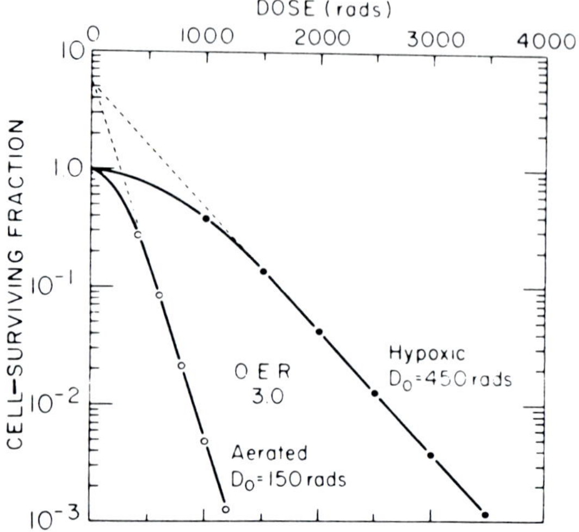

FIG. 2. Survival curves for cultured mammalian (hamster) cells exposed to X-rays under aerated conditions and under hypoxic conditions produced by passing a stream of nitrogen over the cells. At all levels of survival, the dose required to produce a given amount of damage is three times greater under hypoxic conditions. The OER, therefore, is said to be three. (Reproduced with permission from E. J. Hall, *Radiobiology for the Radiologist*, 2nd ed., Harper & Row, 1978.)

the oxygen enhancement ratio (OER) is said to be three. *In vivo*, tumors show similar radioresistance under hypoxic conditions. Experimental radiochemical data suggest that oxygen contributes to radiation lethality by binding to tumor DNA in the zone damaged by the radiation, rendering the damage irreparable.

The role of hypoxia in the radiation therapy of human solid tumors has not been clearly defined. It is probable that resistant hypoxic cells, remaining clonogenic after therapy, could be a barrier to cure. Randomized trials performed in England have produced indirect evidence of hypoxia having detrimental effects on clinical radiation therapy. In these studies of patients with carcinoma of the cervix, the lung, and the head and neck, the survival rate was better for the patients irradiated in an atmosphere of hyperbaric oxygen than it was for those irradiated in a natural environment (12). On the basis of these and other findings, work is being done to evaluate known compounds, and to identify new compounds, that selectively sensitize hypoxic cells to radiation.

The nitroimidazole sensitizers

The nitroimidazoles appear to radiosensitize oxygen-deprived cells by substituting for oxygen in binding to the DNA sites damaged by radiation, making it impossible for the damage to be repaired. These compounds have been a primary focal point in the search for radiosensitizers of hypoxic cells. Metronidazole (Flagy®, Searle), an agent that has already had extensive clinical application as a trichomonacide, and misonidazole (Ro-07-0582), a closely related compound (Fig. 3), are both small molecules with sufficient lipophilicity to cross the blood-brain barrier and penetrate brain tumors with ease. Because the cellular uptake and metabolism of these compounds are much slower than those of oxygen, they should penetrate into the deeper, oxygen-depleted zones of the tumor provided that there is adequate capillary density and blood flow in these deeper tumor regions.

Nitroimidazole sensitization of hypoxic mammalian cells has proved effective in many *in vitro* systems. The presence of misonidazole dramatically decreases the radiation dose necessary to reduce the survival of hypoxic (nitrogen-gassed) cells to a specified level. Because of this ability to sensitize hypoxic cells to radiation *in vitro*, both metronidazole and misonidazole have been tested extensively in several animal tumor models by a variety of methods. One reliable system measures the effect of a sensitizer by its impact on the delay of tumor regrowth caused by radiation. Both compounds retard tumor regrowth in a subcutaneous mouse carcinoma after irradiation, but misonidazole has the more pronounced effect (2,11).

Urtasun et al. selected metronidazole for the first clinical trials of hypoxic cell radiosensitizers in the treatment of human malignancy (56). Glioblastoma multiforme was the object of these trials because of its tendency to aggressive local growth rather than metastasis, and because its partially necrotic character implies a large proportion of hypoxic tumor cells. Patients with glioblastomas were randomized into one group that received radiation therapy only (3,000 rads in nine fractions over 18 days), and another that received radiation therapy with metronidazole (6 g/m^2) administered 4 hours before irradiation. The improvement in the median survival time of patients receiving the metronidazole was statistically significant (Fig. 4), but because the total radiation dose was low, the survival times in both groups were lower than those achieved with a standard radiation regimen.

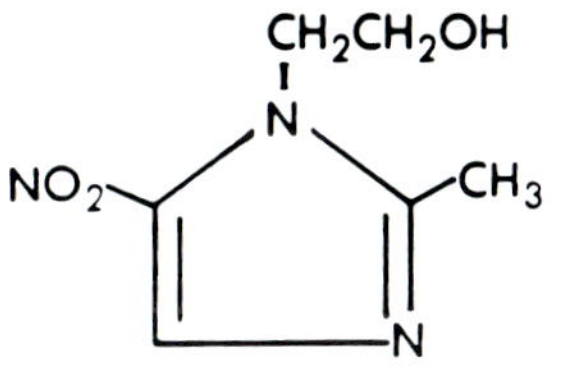

Metronidazole (Flagyl)

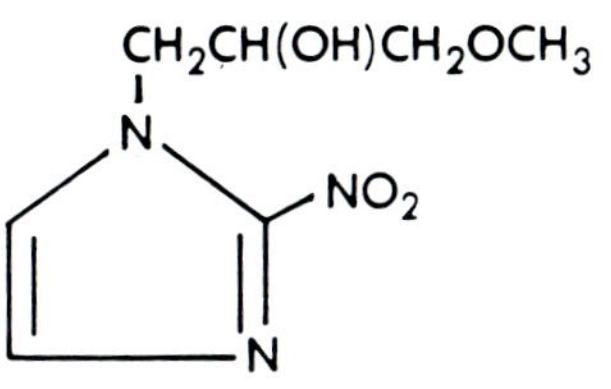

FIG. 3. Structures of metronidazole and misonidazole.

Misonidazole (Ro-07-0582)

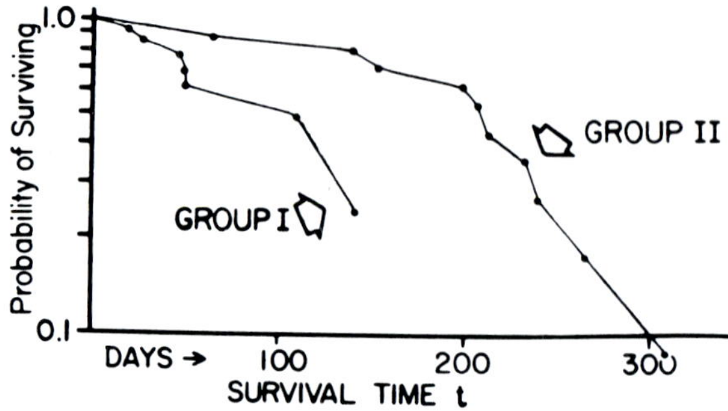

FIG. 4. Probability of survival as a function of time for patients with GM treated either with radiation (3,000 rads in 9 fractions, given 3 times weekly—Group I), or with radiation combined with metronidazole (Group II). (From Urtasun et al., ref. 56, with permission.)

The results of the trial do suggest, however, that a hypoxic cell fraction is present in human brain tumors, and that this cell population influences the tumor's response to irradiation.

Misonidazole, clearly the superior sensitizer in cultured cells and animal systems, is now undergoing extensive clinical testing as a radiosensitizer for solid tumors of all types, including malignant brain tumors, although early results from the large cooperative groups provide no consensus as to its efficacy. What is apparent from these trials, however, is that the drug is toxic. Its principal side effects are nausea, vomiting, and neurotoxicity. Nausea and vomiting occur immediately after a single dose in excess of 5 g/m^2 is ingested; approximately half of the patients treated with lower doses experience nausea and vomiting (63). The manifestation of misonidazole's toxicity that makes dosage restriction imperative is a peripheral (primarily sensory) polyneuropathy characterized by paresthesias and sometimes by impaired proprioception. Encephalopathy, characterized by confusion, coma, and dementia, has occurred in some debilitated, dehydrated patients; muscle weakness and ototoxicity have been observed in rare cases (63).

The neurotoxicity of misonidazole is closely related to the total drug dose rather than to the amount of a single dose. In our experience, the incidence of neuropathy was 21% in patients receiving total doses of less than 10 g/m^2, and 79% in those receiving higher cumulative doses. The time-span over which the total dose was given influenced the incidence of neurotoxicity to some extent; the effect on the peripheral nerves of a cumulative dose of 12 g/m^2 given over a period of 3 weeks was approximately equivalent to that of a cumulative dose of 15 g/m^2 given over 6 weeks (63).

Considering the restrictions on the total dose that can be given safely, various dosage strategies have been proposed (13). The most popular approach is to administer a large dose of sensitizer with high-dose radiation fractions. Another approach is to give the drug with some, but not all, treatments in a conventional fractionated course of radiation therapy; several investigators using this method give the misonidazole and radiation late in the day, and irradiate the patient on the morning of the next day to take advantage of residual misonidazole in the system.

The neuropathies associated with misonidazole are usually nonprogressive and resolve within a short time after use of the drug is discontinued. Neurotoxicity, however, is the serious obstacle. Until hypoxic cell sensitizers are found that are less toxic, these agents must be administered in small, single doses, spaced judiciously over the course of radiation therapy so that the toxic cumulative dose is not exceeded.

Interstitial Radiation

More than 90% of anaplastic astrocytomas and glioblastomas are localized in a single area of the brain (26). These tumors seldom metastasize within the central nervous system (CNS) (15), and systemic metastases are rare (3,52). Most solid tumors that have not metastasized by the time they are detected can be cured by surgery and radiation therapy (66). Nonetheless, investigations into new strategies for the therapy of malignant brain tumors have mainly pursued systemic chemotherapy, a modality more logically suited to disease that spreads beyond its site of origin. Considering the countless obstacles to systemic chemotherapy's efficacy against brain tumors, this emphasis would seem to be misguided.

Among the methods for local therapy of brain tumors that have been proposed are hyperthermia, intratumoral chemotherapy, intra-arterial chemotherapy, and interstitial irradiation. Given the known efficacy of radiation therapy against brain tumors, interstitial irradiation may be the most immediately promising therapeutic approach.

Interstitial radiation has been used for palliative and curative treatment of malignancies at many sites. Because of the relative inaccessibility of brain tumors, however, experience with these lesions is limited—although European neurosurgeons have used stereotactic neurosurgical techniques to successfully implant radioactive sources into brain tumors (53). The increased therapeutic ratio of brachytherapy might permit either delivery of interstitial radiation "boosts" to brain tumors after conventional teletherapy, or the relatively nontoxic interstitial irradiation of previously externally-irradiated recurrent brain tumors. Our experience has been with the stereotactic placement of permanent or removable iridium-192 (^{192}Ir), gold-198 (^{198}Au), and iodine-125 (^{125}I) sources into primary or metastatic brain tumors (22), our recent emphasis being on high-activity ^{125}I.

Implantation technique

Radioactive sources are implanted using the Leksell stereotactic system with the patient under local anesthesia. We have modified the Leksell stereotactic system for use with the General Electric (GE) 8800 CT scanner (38). A base plate is fixed at four points to the outer table of the skull and, with a plastic replica of the conventional metal stereotactic frame attached to the base plate, a CT scan is performed. Scan artifacts that occur with metal frames are avoided, and with the plastic frame in position, the tumor target(s) can be visualized and related precisely to the frame's center by the GE 8800 scanner's integral computer program (Fig.

5). The coordinates for the target sites are calculated, the patient is taken to the operating room, and with the metal frame in position, the radioactive sources are implanted. This method allows us to precisely position the source(s) and perform the implantation in a single operation.

Currently, the source(s) is mounted in a plastic catheter and later removed. Techniques employing a removable implant afford greater control over the dose delivered, prevent migration of the source(s) from necrotic regions of the tumor, and make it possible to remove the source(s) if emergency decompressive surgery is required. In addition, the removable implant system allows the use of long-lived, high-activity ^{125}I, so that the patient can safely return home after treatment and not expose family members to radiation. An afterloaded Silastic® implant catheter[1] is used for placing the removable implants. This catheter affords greater accuracy of placement, and

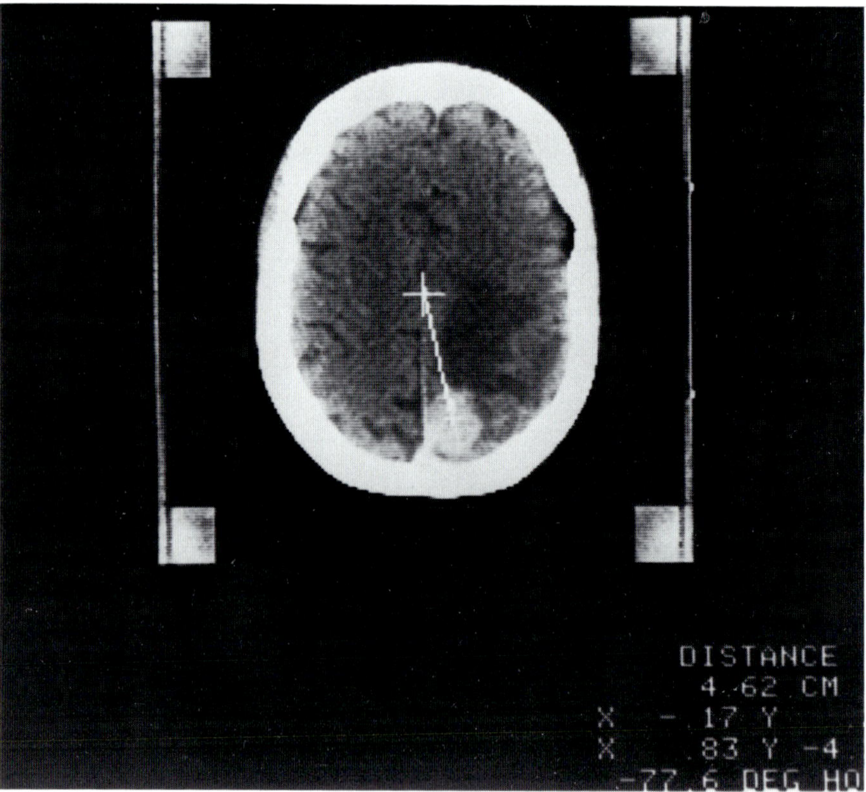

FIG. 5. CT scan taken with the plastic stereotactic frame in position. The four vertical *(square)* posts of the frame are visible. The geometric center of the frame *(small cross)* is related to the target for ^{125}I placement in the tumor by the scanner's computer. The coordinates of the center of the frame and the target are seen at the lower right.

---

[1]Developed in cooperation with the American Heyer-Schulte Corporation, Goleta, California.

radiographic verification of the appropriate position can be obtained before the radioactive sources are placed into the catheter. An outer cannula is passed to the target through the guides of the stereotactic frame and through the interposed brain; after radiographic verification of its position, it is loaded with a coaxial inner cannula containing the source(s). The wound is then reapproximated so the catheter is completely covered.

Removable ^{125}I implants

The recent availability of high-activity ^{125}I sources from the 3M Company (St. Paul, Minnesota) makes it possible to deliver radiation at the dose rate necessary to treat tumors with malignant growth characteristics. Our experience suggests that low-activity ^{125}I sources implanted in reasonable numbers are sufficient only for treating low-grade astrocytomas. Higher activity ^{125}I sources that provide higher radiation dosages per hour are necessary to treat primary or metastatic malignant brain tumors. Dose rates in excess of 30 rad/hr are necessary to treat primary and metastatic malignant brain tumors; equally high dose rates are commonly used in the brachytherapy of cancer at other sites in the body (43).

We have used removable, high-activity ^{125}I implants to treat more than 25 patients harboring primary or metastatic brain tumors. Most of these tumors had recurred after surgery, whole-brain irradiation, and treatment with all feasible chemotherapeutic agents. After receiving interstitial radioactive treatment, nearly all of these patients have shown improvement on CT scans and/or in their clinical status (Fig. 6). Our preliminary results have been reported (22), and we are continuing to refine this technique.

ADJUVANT CHEMOTHERAPY

Cerebral Glioblastoma Multiforme and Anaplastic Astrocytomas

Well-differentiated astrocytomas usually cannot be resected because of their infiltration of the normal brain. In general, these tumors grow much more slowly than the anaplastic astrocytomas and glioblastomas. Since they often respond to radiation alone (49), we do not use adjuvant chemotherapy.

Most of the rapidly growing anaplastic astrocytomas and glioblastomas are confirmed by surgery and subtotally removed. They are moderately responsive to radiation therapy. The best known postoperative treatment for these tumors involves, at the minimum, irradiation of the tumor to a dose of 6,000 rads, together with whole-brain irradiation of 4,500 to 5,000 rads; and concomitant adjuvant chemotherapy with 1,3-*bis*(2-chloroethyl)-1-nitrosourea (BCNU), either 80 mg/m^2 daily for 3 days, or 220 mg/m^2 daily for 1 day, before radiation therapy is instituted and at 6 to 8-week intervals thereafter. This regimen of adjuvant chemotherapy produces an increase in the mean time to tumor progression (MTP), and the number of long-term survivors is greater than is achieved with radiation therapy alone (60).

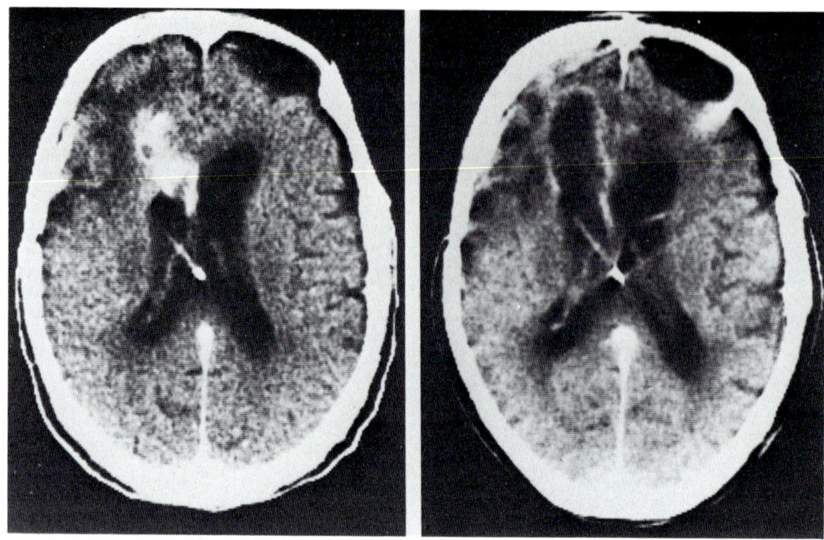

FIG. 6. CT scan showing a right frontal glioblastoma before *(left)* and 2 months after *(right)* treatment with removable implanted sources of high-activity ^{125}I.

TABLE 1. *Time to tumor progression and survival for patients with glioblastoma multiforme (GM)*

Therapy	No. of patients	MTP (weeks)	Median survival (weeks)	Reference
BCNU − RT	45		40[a]	Walker et al. (60)
BCNU + RT	26	31[b]	50[b]	Levin et al. (36)
BCNU + HU + RT	35	42[b]	57[b]	Levin et al. (37)
RT + HU + BCNU	36	36[b]	49[b]	NCOG statistical report (42)
RT + HU + PCV	30	37[b]	42[b]	NCOG statistical report (42)
BCNU + RT	92		51[c]	Walker et al. (61)

MTP = median time to tumor progression; RT = radiation therapy; HU = hydroxyurea; PCV = procarbazine + CCNU + vincristine combination.
[a]90% GM, 10% NGM (only patients receiving two courses of BCNU included).
[b]GM only.
[c]81% GM, 19% NGM.

For treating glioblastoma multiforme, the addition of hydroxyurea (HU), 275 mg/m² every 6 hours every other day during irradiation, to the BCNU schedule further increases the MTP and adds to long-term survival (36). For anaplastic astrocytomas, the addition of HU does not appear to offer any substantial benefit.

The data available through 1980 on the MTP and survival of patients in six reasonably similar adjuvant chemotherapy programs are summarized in Table 1.

Procarbazine (150 mg/m^2 per day $\times$ 28), administered during radiation therapy and at 8-week intervals thereafter, appears to be nearly as effective as BCNU in increasing the MTP (59). No other adjuvant chemotherapy program with single agents has proved to be more effective than BCNU or procarbazine (32,59), although these agents are by no means optimally effective.

Brain Stem Astrocytomas

For most brain stem gliomas, the clinical features and neuroradiological studies usually establish an unequivocal diagnosis. When the clinical picture is atypical, when radiological studies indicate an exophytic (extra-axial) mass, or when a cystic mass is suspected (usually on the basis of CT scans), surgical exploration is indicated.

Even with radiation therapy, the course of this disease is a steady progression to death, with a median survival of 4 to 15 months (1,50), although in some patients the course of the disease may be more indolent. Several studies show a correlation between the prognosis and the location or pathology of the tumor: tumors of the upper pons and midbrain are likely to be well-differentiated astrocytomas, whereas those of the lower pons and medulla are more likely to be malignant (45).

The role of adjuvant chemotherapy in the treatment of brain stem astrocytomas has not been well established. A recent appraisal of these tumors by the Childrens Cancer Study Group (CCSG protocol 944) compared the results of irradiation (5,000 to 6,000 rads) to those of irradiation administered together with the combination of 1-(2-chloroethyl)-3-cyclohexyl-1-nitrosourea (CCNU) and vincristine; 38% of the children in the former group, and 55% of those in the latter, were alive at 1 year after the diagnosis was established (9). In a series of patients recently reported by Fulton et al. (19), the median survival was 45 weeks for patients who received chemotherapy adjuvant to radiation therapy, whereas it was 56 weeks for patients who received no chemotherapy until after the tumor recurred following a course of radiation therapy. In the two groups, the 1-year survival was 8% and 65%, respectively.

Medulloblastoma

Among patients with this highly radiosensitive tumor, craniospinal irradiation results in approximately 30% survival at 10 years (5,6,50). Recently, studies evaluating adjuvant chemotherapy were initiated by the Société Internationale Oncologie Pediatrique (SIOP) and the CCSG. The adjuvant chemotherapy program in the SIOP study consisted of CCNU and vincristine; the program in the CCSG study consisted of CCNU, vincristine, and prednisone. In the CCSG study, there was no difference between the results achieved with radiation therapy only and those achieved with irradiation and chemotherapy, whereas in the SIOP study there was a difference in favor of the chemotherapy arm. However, the results achieved in the chemotherapy arm of the SIOP study were no better than those achieved in the irradiation only arm of the CCSG study (9,16). We evaluated the results obtained with an adjuvant regimen of procarbazine, CCNU, and vincristine (PCV) in a small series of 7 patients who had undergone surgery and radiation therapy. In 6-week cycles they received CCNU, day 1, 45 mg/m²; procarbazine, days 8–29, 60 mg/m²; and vincristine, days 8 and 29, 1.4 mg/m². The addition of this PCV2 regimen offered no benefit over therapy with surgery and irradiation alone (unpublished observation). Venes et al. (57) studied 8 children who received a vincristine-cyclophosphamide combination following radiation therapy; the median follow-up at 4 years showed no recurrence of tumor.

These last two series are too small to permit conclusions. At this juncture, the benefit of adjuvant chemotherapy is anticipated, but its overall efficacy remains unproved. The main problem in any chemotherapy program for medulloblastoma is that craniospinal radiation reduces the patient's ability to tolerate myelosuppressive chemotherapy. In designing future adjuvant chemotherapy programs, a pivotal issue will be a reduction in the dose of spinal radiation (to less than 2,500 rads when myelography is negative) to allow more aggressive chemotherapy during and after radiation.

Metastatic Tumors

Tumors metastatic to the CNS account for nearly 50% of brain tumors. The incidence varies from hospital to hospital but, in general, carcinoma of the lung, carcinoma of the breast, and melanoma represent the three most common groups of tumors metastasizing to the CNS.

As a rule, the likelihood of metastases to the CNS increases in proportion to the duration of systemic disease and with the presence of pulmonary metastases. Surgery and irradiation are palliative treatments, seldom affording more than 3 to 8 months of survival. Tables 2, 3, and 4 summarize results that are typical in cases of CNS metastases. There is little data on the adjuvant chemotherapy of these tumors.

A few solitary metastatic brain tumors that arise from an occult primary source are mistaken for primary tumors, and are treated surgically. Occasionally, metastatic tumors are resected for the purpose of "cure," presuming that the brain metastasis represents the only metastatic lesion, or for surgical decompression to relieve impending transtentorial herniation. With few exceptions, operative removal should

TABLE 2. *Survival for patients with brain metastases: lung*

Tumor type	Incidence (%)	Median survival (months)
Small cell	30	4.1
Large cell	29	>5.4
Adenocarcinoma	25	4.8
Epidermoid	14	2.4

Data from Newman and Hansen, ref. 40.

TABLE 3. *Benefit of treatment (surgery and/or irradiation) for 82 "good" risk patients with single brain lesions, no metastatic disease outside the CNS, and squamous cell carcinoma or adenocarcinoma*

Treatment	Median survival (months)
No treatment	2.1
Surgery	6.5
Irradiation	5.5
Surgery and irradiation	6.0

Data from McGuire et al., ref. 39.

TABLE 4. *Response to treatment in patients with brain metastases: melanoma*

Treatment	No. of patients	Mean survival (months)
No treatment	19	0.9
Surgery	4	22.0
Irradiation	16	4.0
Chemotherapy	17	2.2
Only CNS metastases		7.5
CNS and visceral metastases		<1.0

Data from Amer et al., ref. 4.

be followed by whole-brain irradiation, even though it is only palliative in most cases. Because of the diversity of tumors metastasizing to the brain and the frequent need to continue chemotherapy for systemic or primary tumor control, few adjuvant chemotherapy programs have been designed for brain metastases.

RECURRENT TUMORS

Recurrent tumors are those that either fail to respond to, or recur after, primary treatment by operation, irradiation, and chemotherapy, either individually or in combination.

Cerebral Glioblastoma Multiforme and Anaplastic Astrocytomas

BCNU, CCNU, and procarbazine used as single agents against recurrent cerebral glioblastoma multiforme and anaplastic astrocytomas have produced comparable response rates (7,35,65) (Table 5). To enhance the efficacy of BCNU, we developed a protocol in which 5-fluorouracil (FU) was given 2 weeks after BCNU administration, at a time when tumor cell repopulation was calculated to be maximal. This combination of drugs temporarily arrested disease progression in 83% of patients by producing either improvement or stability (34). There was a dose-response

TABLE 5. *Response to treatment in patients with supratentorial malignant gliomas*

Agent	% Improved (R + S/total)	MTP (weeks)	Reference
BCNU	50 (20/40)[a]	38/—[c]	Wilson et al. (64)
			Levin and Wilson (35)
CCNU	45 (10/22)[c]	24/—[c]	Fewer et al. (18)
PCB	50 (10/20)[c]	26/—[c]	Kumar et al. (29)
			Levin and Wilson (35)
MeCCNU	28 (8/29)[c]	44/—[d]	Tranum et al. (55)
BCNU-VCR	50 (6/12)	17/—	Fewer et al. (17)
BCNU-PCB	40 (21/52)	34/20	Levin et al. (31)
BCNU-FU	83 (24/29)	34/26	Levin et al. (34)
BCNU-FU-HU-6MP	67 (10/15)	38/22	Levin et al., unpublished observations
CCNU-PCB-VCR (PCV1)	62 (18/29)	30/—	Gutin et al. (23)
CCNU-PCB-VCR (PCV3)	84 (16/19)	31/25	Levin et al. (33)
CCNU-PCB-VCR (PCV3)	44 (12/27)[b]		Levin et al. (33)

Data adapted from ref. 30, Levin's nitrosoureas study.

R + S = response + stable disease patients; MTP = median time to tumor progression; PCB = procarbazine; MeCCNU = methyl-CCNU; VCR = vincristine; FU = 5-fluorouracil; HU = hydroxyurea; 6MP = mercaptopurine; PCV = procarbazine + CCNU + vincristine.

[a]Responders and stable disease patients combined. No previous chemotherapy given to patients in these studies.

[b]Previous chemotherapy.

[c]These values are overestimated because previous response criteria required clinical deterioration together with RN scan evidence of tumor enlargement.

[d]Criteria of response not comparable to other studies.

relationship, in that patients who were designated "responders" tolerated higher dosages of BCNU during their first five courses of chemotherapy than did those who were designated in the category of "stabilized disease." The MTP for the entire group was 26 weeks, and that for the responders was 34 weeks. Only 17% of patients were alive at the end of 1 year (Table 5).

In an effort to improve on this therapy, we added HU and 6-mercaptopurine (6MP) to the BCNU-FU combination. A preliminary analysis of the data from 34 patients shows no significant difference between BCNU-FU and the new combination of BCNU-FU-HU-6MP (unpublished observation).

Combinations of CCNU and procarbazine, either with or without vincristine added, have been effective against a number of CNS tumors. Our scheduling of PCV for patients with recurrent gliomas has changed over the years (PCV1, PCV3). From the results of animal studies, we have reduced systemic toxicity by instituting treatment with procarbazine 1 week after the initiation of therapy with CCNU and by reducing the dosage of procarbazine: 6-week cycles of CCNU, day 1, 110 mg/m^2; procarbazine, days 8–29, 60 mg/m^2; and vincristine, days 8 and 29, 1.4 mg/m^2. Unlike the study of the BCNU-FU combination, this PCV3 protocol was evaluated in a mixed patient population, among whom 59% had received prior chemotherapy (33). Of the patients who had not received prior chemotherapy, 42% responded, and in 42% the disease stabilized; whereas among patients who had received prior chemotherapy, only 15% responded, and 30% had stabilization of disease. We were interested to find that, among patients who showed either response or disease stabilization, the MTP differed little between those who had received prior chemotherapy and those who had not; the MTP was 27 weeks, and 30% of patients were alive at 1 year.

In both the PCV3 and BCNU-FU studies, patients with glioblastoma multiforme invariably did considerably worse (MTP, approximately 12 to 14 weeks) than those who had nonglioblastoma malignant glioma (MTP, 26 to 27 weeks). The most important feature in common between the BCNU-FU and PCV3 combinations is an ability to halt disease progression; unfortunately, long-term remission was not achieved by the new programs when the results were compared, respectively, to those with either BCNU alone (64) or PCV1 (23).

Brain Stem Tumors

Because the histology of brain stem tumors is similar to those of cerebral glioblastoma multiforme and anaplastic astrocytomas, theoretically they should respond to the same oncolytic agents. But the results of chemotherapeutic treatment of recurrent brain stem tumors have been disappointing with respect to both the frequency and duration of response (19). In 24 of our patients who received radiation therapy after initial diagnosis, chemotherapy was given when tumor progression was first diagnosed. They either received CCNU, BCNU, or procarbazine alone, or were given a combination of: (a) CCNU, FU, HU, and 6MP, or (b) CCNU and procarbazine, or (c) BCNU and procarbazine. The MTP was 34 weeks; the median survival was 56 weeks. It seemed to be of little consequence whether the drug schedules and combinations used in the program were nitrosourea-prominent or procarbazine-prominent: these patients did badly.

Medulloblastoma

Various chemotherapeutic agents can be used to palliate medulloblastoma at the time of recurrence. The combinations of procarbazine, CCNU, and vincristine (10); of vincristine, methotrexate, and cyclophosphamide (24); and of vincristine, BCNU, and methotrexate (14); as well as single-agent programs with procarbazine (29), intrathecal methotrexate (41), vincristine (47,51) or oral dibromodulcitol (DBD) (unpublished observations) have shown some antitumor activity. Nevertheless, since prior craniospinal irradiation irreversibly damages bone marrow stem cells, chemotherapeutic efforts to treat recurrent tumors are compromised; this is one reason that chemotherapy for medulloblastoma recurrence is only palliative.

Recurrent medulloblastoma may also be treated by a second course of radiation therapy, administration either alone or in conjunction with either a nitroimidazole radiosensitizer such as misonidazole, which is currently being used in a study by the Radiation Therapy Oncology Group (RTOG) and the CCSG, or with a radiopotentiator such as HU. The preliminary results of the RTOG-CCSG study suggest that the levels of palliation achieved with these programs are similar to those achieved with chemotherapy, but it is too early to assess the long-term toxic effects of reirradiation on the CNS (W. Wara, personal communication, 1980).

We recently reviewed the results achieved in 35 of our patients with recurrent medulloblastoma who received aggressive sequential multiple systemic and intrathecal chemotherapy and, in many cases, reirradiation supplemented by misonidazole. The median survival was 2.5 years, and the 25th quartile survival was 3.5 years. We conclude that the potential for effecting long-term palliation, and in a number of cases a cure, does exist—in the treatment of recurrent medulloblastoma to a greater extent than in that of any other recurrent malignant brain tumor.

Metastatic Tumors

Chemotherapy produces no better results in recurrent metastatic tumors than in recurrent gliomas. Tables 6 to 8 summarize studies from the literature regarding metastases from the lung and breast and from melanoma. In addition to the regimens cited in Tables 6 to 8, breast tumors metastatic to the brain respond to thiotepa (21), BCNU, CCNU, and the combination of BCNU-FU (unpublished observations). Reticulum cell sarcoma (microglioma, diffuse histiocytic lymphoma), pri-

TABLE 6. *Response to treatment in patients with brain metastases: lung*

Treatment	% Improved	Survival (months)	Reference
BCNU-RT	25 (5/20)	4.0 (median)	Robusteilli et al. (46)
CCNU-RT	21 (5/24)	4.5 (median)	Robusteilli et al. (46)
CCNU-VCR-MTX	5 (1/20)	1.0 (median)[a]	Hildebrand et al. (25)
CCNU-ADR-RT	36 (8/22)	8.0 (median)[b]	Chan and Byfield (8)
CCNU-ADR-VM 26	23 (3/13)	2.4 (mean)	Pouillart et al. (44)

RT = radiation therapy; VCR = vincristine; MTX = methotrexate; ADR = adriamycin; VM 26 = epipodophyllotoxin.
[a]Patients failed 19/20.
[b]Only 2/14 died of brain metastases.

TABLE 7. *Response to treatment in patients with brain metastases: breast*

Treatment	% Improved	Survival (months)	Reference
CCNU-VCR-MTX	45 (5/11)	8 (mean)	Hildebrand et al. (25)
CCNU-VM 26-ADR	75 (6/8)	8 (mean)	Pouillart et al. (44)
CCNU-RT	50 (7/14)	7 (median)	Robusteilli et al. (46)
BCNU-RT	54 (7/13)	8 (median)	Robusteilli et al. (46)
CYT-FU-PRED	63 (17/27)	7 (median)	Rosner and Nemoto (48)
CYT-FU-PRED-MTX-VCR	61 (8/13)	7 (median)	Rosner and Nemoto (48)
CYT-MNU	44 (4/9)	11 (median)	Kolaric and Roth (28)

RT = radiation therapy; VCR = vincristine; MTX = methotrexate; VM 26 = epipodophyllotoxin; ADR = adriamycin; FU = 5-fluorouracil; PRED = prednisone; CYT-MNU = cyclophosphamide-methyl nitrosourea.

TABLE 8. *Response to treatment in patients with brain metastases: melanoma*

Treatment	% Improved	Survival (months)	Reference
BCNU-RT	67 (4/6)	5 (median)	Robusteilli et al. (46)
CCNU-RT	50 (4/8)	6 (median)	Robusteilli et al. (46)
CYT-MNU	50 (5/10)	9 (median)	Kolaric and Roth (28)

RT = radiation therapy; CYT-MNU = cyclophosphamide-methyl nitrosourea.

mary in or metastatic to the brain, responds to PCV3 (unpublished observations). Responses of melanoma have also been seen to occur with PCV3 and the combination of BCNU and vincristine (18). In some cases of small cell carcinoma, PCV3 is effective. In all cases, the effects of chemotherapy have resulted in short-term palliation; the systemic disease is frequently (in approximately 65% of cases) responsible for death.

ACKNOWLEDGMENTS

This work was supported in part by Department of Health, Education and Welfare Program Project CA-13525, and by American Cancer Society Junior Faculty Clinical Fellowship 557 (P.H.G.), and American Cancer Society Faculty Research Award 155 (V.A.L.). The authors gratefully acknowledge the assistance of Susan Eastwood in the editorial development of the chapter, and of Beverly Hunter in the preparation of the manuscript.

REFERENCES

1. Abramson, N., Raben, M., and Cavanaugh, P. J. (1974): Brain tumors in children: Analysis of 136 cases. *Radiology*, 112:669–672.
2. Adams, G. E., Flockhart, I. R., Smithen, C. E., Stratford, I. J., Wardman, P., and Watts, M. E. (1976): Electron-affinic sensitization: VII. A correlation between structures, one-electron reduction potentials, and efficiencies of nitroimidazoles as hypoxic cell radiosensitizers. *Radiat. Res.*, 67:9–20.
3. Alvord, E. C. (1976): Why do gliomas not metastasize? *Arch. Neurol.*, 33:73–75.
4. Amer, M. H., Al-Sarraf, M., Baker, L. H., and Vaitkevicius, V. K. (1978): Malignant melanoma and central nervous system metastases. *Cancer*, 42:660–668.
5. Bloom, H. J. G. (1971): Concepts in the natural history and treatment of medulloblastoma in children. *CRC Crit. Rev. Radiol. Sci.*, 2:89–143.
6. Bloom, H. J. G., Wallace, E. N. K., and Henk, J. M. (1969): The treatment and prognosis of medulloblastoma in children. A study of 82 verified cases. *Am. J. Roentgenol.*, 105:43–62.
7. Broder, L. E., and Rall, D. P. (1972): Chemotherapy of brain tumors. *Prog. Exp. Tumor Res.*, 17:373–399.
8. Chan, P. Y., and Byfield, J. E. (1979): Adriamycin (AD), CCNU, and X-ray therapy (XRT) in the treatment of brain metastasis (BM) from lung cancer (Meeting abstract). *Int. J. Radiat. Oncol. Biol. Phys. (Suppl.1)*, 5:33.
9. Childrens Cancer Study Group (1981): CCSG Progress Report (February). Los Angeles, California.
10. Crafts, D. C., Levin, V. A., Edwards, M. S., Pischer, T. L., and Wilson, C. B. (1978): Chemotherapy of recurrent medulloblastoma with combined procarbazine, CCNU and vincristine. *J. Neurosurg.*, 49:589–592.
11. Denekamp, J., and Harris, S. R. (1975): Tests of two electron-affinic radiosensitizers *in vivo* using regrowth of an experimental carcinoma. *Radiat. Res.*, 61:191–203.

12. Dische, S. (1978): Hyperbaric oxygen: The Medical Research Council trials and their clinical significance. *Br. J. Radiol.*, 51:888–894.
13. Dische, S., Saunders, M. I., and Flockhart, I. R. (1978): The optimum regime for the administration of misonidazole and the establishment of multi-centre clinical trials. *Br. J. Cancer (Suppl. III)*, 37:318–321.
14. Duffner, P. K., Cohen, M. E., Thomas, P. R. M., Sinks, L., and Freeman, A. I. (1979): Combination chemotherapy in recurrent medulloblastoma. *Cancer*, 43:41–45.
15. Erlich, S. S., and Davis, R. L. (1978): Spinal subarachnoid metastasis from primary intracranial glioblastoma multiforme. *Cancer*, 42:2854–2864.
16. Evans, A. E., Anderson, J., Chang, C., Jenkin, R. D. T., Kramer, S., Schoenfeld, D., and Wilson, C. B. (1979): Adjuvant chemotherapy for medulloblastoma and ependymoma. In: *Multidisciplinary Aspects of Brain Tumor Therapy*, edited by P. Paoletti, M. D. Walker, G. Butti, and R. Knerich, pp. 219–222. Elsevier/North-Holland Biomedical Press, Amsterdam.
17. Fewer, D., Wilson, C. B., Boldrey, E. B., and Enot, K. J. (1972a): A phase II study of 1-(2-chloroethyl)-3-cyclohexyl-1-nitrosourea (CCNU). *Cancer Chemother. Rep.*, 56:421–427.
18. Fewer, D., Wilson, C. B., Boldrey, E. B., Enot, K. J., and Powell, M. R. (1972b): The chemotherapy of brain tumors. Clinical experience with carmustine (BCNU) and vincristine. *J.A.M.A.*, 222:549–552.
19. Fulton, D. S., Levin, V. A., and Wilson, C. B. (1980): Chemotherapy of pediatric brain stem tumors. *J. Neurosurg.*, 54:721–725.
20. Gray, L. H., Conger, A. D., Ebert, M., Hornsey, S., and Scott, O. C. A. (1953): The concentration of oxygen dissolved in tissues at the time of irradiation as a factor in radiotherapy. *Br. J. Radiol.*, 26:638–648.
21. Greenspan, E. M. (1966): Combination cytotoxic chemotherapy in advanced disseminated breast carcinoma. *Mt. Sinai J. Med.*, 33:1–27.
22. Gutin, P. H., Phillips, T. L., Hosobuchi, Y., Wara, W. M., MacKay, A. R., Weaver, K. A., Lamb, S., and Hurst, S. (1981): Permanent and removable implants for the brachytherapy of brain tumors. *Int. J. Radiat. Oncol. Biol. Phys.*, 7:1371–1381.
23. Gutin, P. H., Wilson, C. B., Kumar, A. R. V., Boldrey, E. B., Levin, V. A., Powell, M., and Enot, K. J. (1975): Phase II study of procarbazine, CCNU, and vincristine combination chemotherapy in the treatment of malignant brain tumors. *Cancer*, 35:1398–1404.
24. Hagler, S., Currimbhoy, Z. E., and Tinsley, M. (1968): Cerebellar medulloblastoma. Chemotherapeutic remission with vincristine, cyclophosphamide, and methotrexate. *Cancer*, 21:912–919.
25. Hildebrand, J., Brihaye, J., Wagenkneecht, L., Michel, J., and Kenis, Y. (1975): Combination chemotherapy with CCNU, vincristine, and methotrexate in primary and metastatic brain tumors. *Eur. J. Cancer*, 11:585–587.
26. Hochberg, F. H., and Pruitt, A. (1980): Assumptions in the radiotherapy of glioblastoma. *Neurology*, 30:907–911.
27. Holthusen, H. (1921): Beitrage zur Biologie der Strahlenwirkung. *Pfluegers Arch.*, 187:1–24.
28. Kolaric, K., and Roth, A. (1980): Treatment of metastatic brain tumors with the combination of 1-methyl-1-nitrosourea (MNU) and cyclophosphamide. *J. Cancer Res. Clin. Oncol.*, 97:193–198.
29. Kumar, A. R. V., Renaudin, C., Wilson, C. B., Boldrey, E. B., Enot, K. J., and Levin, V. A. (1974): Procarbazine hydrochloride in the treatment of brain tumors. *J. Neurosurg.*, 40:365–371.
30. Levin, V. A. (1981): Chemotherapy of recurrent brain tumors. In: *Nitrosoureas: Current Status and New Developments*, edited by A. W. Prestayko, L. H. Baker, S. T. Crooke, S. K. Carter, and P. S. Schein, pp. 259–267. Academic Press, New York.
31. Levin, V. A., Crafts, D. C., Wilson, C. B., Schultz, M. J., Boldrey, E. B., Enot, K. J., Pischer, T. L., Seager, M., and Elashoff, R. M. (1976): BCNU and procarbazine treatment for malignant brain tumors. *Cancer Treat. Rep.*, 60:243–249.
32. Levin, V. A., and Edwards, M. S. (1980): Chemotherapy of primary malignant gliomas. In: *Brain Tumors: Scientific Basis, Clinical Investigation, and Current Therapy*, edited by D. G. T. Thomas and D. Graham, pp. 344–358. Butterworths, London.
33. Levin, V. A., Edwards, M. S., Wright, D. C., Seager, M. L., Pischer, T. L., Townsend, J., and Wilson, C. B. (1980): Modified procarbazine, CCNU and vincristine combination chemotherapy (UCSF PCV3) in the treatment of malignant brain tumors. *Cancer Treat. Rep.*, 64:237–241.
34. Levin, V. A., Hoffman, W. F., Pischer, T. L., Seager, M. L., Boldrey, E. B., and Wilson, C. B. (1978): BCNU-5-fluorouracil combination therapy for recurrent malignant brain tumors. *Cancer Treat. Rep.*, 62:2071–2076.

35. Levin, V. A., and Wilson, C. B. (1975): Chemotherapy: Agents in current use. *Semin. Oncol.*, 2:63–68.
36. Levin, V. A., Wilson, C. B., Davis, R., Wara, W., Pischer, T. L., and Irwin, L. (1979*a*): A phase III comparison of BCNU, hydroxyurea, and radiation therapy to BCNU and radiation therapy for treatment of primary malignant gliomas. *J. Neurosurg.*, 51:526–532.
37. Levin, V. A., Wilson, C. B., Davis, R., Wara, W., Pischer, T. L., and Irwin, L. (1979*b*): Preliminary results of a phase III comparison study of BCNU, hydroxyurea, and radiation to BCNU and radiation. *Int. J. Radiat. Oncol. Biol. Phys.*, 5:1573–1576.
38. MacKay, A., Gutin, P., Hosobuchi, Y., and Norman, D. (1981): CT stereotaxis and interstitial radiation for brain tumor. In: *Interventional Radiologic Techniques: Computerized Tomography and Ultrasonography*, edited by A. A. Moss and H. I. Goldberg, pp. 93–99. University of California Printing Department, San Francisco.
39. McGuire, T. J., Smith, S. B., Kerby, G. R., and Fixley, M. S. (1979): Survival of patients with lung carcinoma metastatic to the brain: Comparison of therapies (Meeting Abstract). *Proc. Am. Assoc. Cancer Res.*, 20:393.
40. Newman, S. J., and Hansen, H. H. (1974): Frequency, diagnosis, and treatment of brain metastases in 247 consecutive patients with bronchogenic carcinoma. *Cancer*, 33:492–496.
41. Newton, W. A., Sayers, M. P., and Samuels, L. D. (1968): Intrathecal methotrexate therapy for brain tumors in children. *Cancer Chemother. Rep.*, 52:257–261.
42. Northern California Oncology Group (1980): NCOG Statistical Report (October). Palo Alto, California.
43. Pierquin, B. (1976): The destiny of brachytherapy in oncology. *Am. J. Roentgenol.*, 127:495–499.
44. Pouillart, P., Mathe, G., Thy, T. H., Lheritier, J., Poisson, M., Huguenin, P., Gauthier, H., Morin, P., and Parrot, R. (1976): Treatment of malignant gliomas and brain metastases in adults with a combination of adriamycin, VM 26, and CCNU: Results of a phase II trial. *Cancer*, 38:1909–1916.
45. Reigel, D. H., Scarff, T. B., and Woodford, J. E. (1979): The biopsy of pediatric brain stem tumors. *Childs Brain*, 5:329–340.
46. Robusteilli Della Luna, G. R., Paoletti, P., Bertolotti, E., Knerick, R., Bernadinelli, L., Butti, G., and Baldi, M. (1979): Combined modality treatment of metastatic central nervous system (CNS) tumors with nitrosourea compounds. In: *Multidisciplinary Aspects of Brain Tumor Therapy*, edited by P. Paoletti, M. D. Walker, G. Butti, and R. Knerich, pp. 283–298. Elsevier, Amsterdam.
47. Rosenstock, J. G., Evans, A. E., and Schut, L. (1976): Response to vincristine of recurrent brain tumors in children. *J. Neurosurg.*, 45:135–140.
48. Rosner, D., and Nemoto, T. (1980): Combination chemotherapy of brain metastasis in breast cancer (Meeting Abstract). *Proc. Am. Assoc. Cancer Res.*, 21:405.
49. Sheline, G. E. (1975*a*): Radiation therapy of primary tumors. *Semin. Oncol.*, 2:29–42.
50. Sheline, G. E. (1975*b*): Radiation therapy of tumors of the central nervous system in childhood. *Cancer*, 35:957–964.
51. Smart, C. R., Ottoman, R. E., Rochlin, D. B., Hornes, D. B., Sylva, J., Antonio, R., and Goepfert, H. (1968): Clinical experience with vincristine (NSC-67574) in tumors of the central nervous system and other malignant diseases. *Cancer Chemother. Rep.*, 52:733–741.
52. Smith, D. R., Hardman, K. M., and Earle, K. M. (1969): Metastasizing neuroectodermal tumors of the central nervous system. *J. Neurosurg.*, 31:50–58.
53. Szikla, G., editor (1979): *Stereotactic Cerebral Irradiation*. Biomedical Press, Elsevier/North-Holland, Amsterdam.
54. Thomlinson, R. H., and Gray, L. H. (1955): The histological structure of some human lung cancers and the possible implications of radiotherapy. *Br. J. Cancer*, 9:539–549.
55. Tranum, B. L., Haut, A., Rivkin, S., Weber, E., Quagliana, J. M., Shaw, M., Tucker, W. G., Smith, F. E., Samson, M., and Gottlieb, J. (1975): A phase II study of methyl CCNU in the treatment of solid tumors and lymphomas: A Southwest Oncology Group study. *Cancer*, 35:1148–1153.
56. Urtasun, R. C., Band, P., Chapman, J. D., Feldstein, M. L., Mielke, B., and Fryer, C. (1976): Radiation and high-dose metronidazole in supratentorial glioblastomas. *N. Engl. J. Med.*, 294:1364–1367.
57. Venes, J. L., McIntosh, S., O'Brien, R. T., and Schwartz, A. D. (1979): Chemotherapy as an adjunct in the initial management of cerebellar medulloblastomas. A preliminary report. *J. Neurosurg.*, 50:721–724.

58. Walker, M. D. (1975): Chemotherapy: Adjuvant to surgery and radiation therapy. *Semin. Oncol.*, 2:69–72.
59. Walker, M. D. (1981): Brain Tumor Study Group: Clinical Trials. (Proc. 3rd Conf. Brain Tumor Therapy, October 1979). *Cancer Treat. Rep. (in press).*
60. Walker, M. D., Alexander, E., Jr., Hunt, W. E., MacCarty, C. S., Mahaley, M. S., Jr., Mealey, J., Norrell, H. A., Owens, G., Ransohoff, J., Wilson, C. B., Gehan, E. A., and Strike, T. A. (1978): Evaluation of BCNU and/or radiotherapy in the treatment of anaplastic gliomas. A cooperative clinical trial. *J. Neurosurg.*, 49:333–343.
61. Walker, M. D., Green, S. B., Byar, D. P., Alexander, E., Batzdorf, U., Brooks, W. H., Hunt, W. E., MacCarty, C. S. Mahaley, M. S., Mealey, J., Owens, G., Ransohoff, J., Robertson, J. T., Shapiro, W. R., Smith, K. R., Wilson, C. B., and Strike, T. A. (1980): Randomized comparisons of radiotherapy and nitrosoureas for the treatment of malignant glioma after surgery. *N. Engl. J. Med.*, 303:1323–1329.
62. Walker, M. D., Strike, T. A., and Sheline, G. E. (1979): An analysis of dose-effect relationship in the radiotherapy of malignant gliomas. *Int. J. Radiat. Oncol. Biol. Phys.*, 5:1733–1740.
63. Wasserman, T. H., Phillips, T. L., Johnson, R. J., Gomer, C. J., Lawrence, G. A., Sadee, W., and VanRaalte, G. (1979): Initial United States clinical pharmacologic evaluation of misonidazole (Ro-07-0582), an hypoxic cell radiosensitizer. *Int. J. Radiat. Oncol. Biol. Phys.*, 5:775–786.
64. Wilson, C. B., Boldrey, E. B., and Enot, K. J. (1970): 3-*bis*-(2-chloroethyl)-1-nitrosourea (NSC-409962) in the treatment of brain tumors. *Cancer Chemother. Rep.*, 54:273–281.
65. Wilson, C. B., Gutin, P. H., Boldrey, E. B., Crafts, D. C., Levin, V. A., and Enot, K. J. (1976): Single-agent chemotherapy of brain tumors: A five-year review. *Arch. Neurol.*, 33:739–744.
66. Zubrod, C. G. (1972): Chemical control of cancer. *Proc. Natl. Acad. Sci. USA*, 69:1042–1047.

Controversies in Neurology, edited by R. A. Thompson and J. R. Green. Raven Press, New York © 1983.

Indications and Techniques for Biopsy for Treatment Planning

Russel H. Patterson, Jr.

525 East 68th Street, New York, New York 10021

Those of us who deal with brain tumor at the Cornell Medical Center, which includes The New York Hospital and the Memorial Sloan-Kettering Cancer Institute, have developed a bias toward obtaining tissue from all patients with undiagnosed intracranial mass lesions. Our experience, which now is about 300 operated cases of brain tumor annually, has shown that this can be accomplished safely most of the time. Brain stem gliomas are a possible exception, but in recent years even most of them have been biopsied. Some cases presented below illustrate this point, and make a few others that we have come to believe are important in setting the stage for subsequent therapy.

LESIONS OF THE BRAIN STEM

Case 1. S. B., a 9-year-old child, proved to have a straightforward brain stem glioma, but her case illustrates that cystic or exophytic masses in the brain stem are, for the most part, amenable to biopsy.

Seven months prior to surgery, S. B. developed headaches of increasing severity that were treated as migraine until 1 month prior to admission when the child developed neck pain, double vision, head tilt, and a left hemiparesis. A CT scan, lumbar puncture, myelogram, and angiogram were normal except for an elevated cerebrospinal fluid (CSF) protein. The administration of corticosteroids helped, but when the dosage was reduced, headache increased and dysuria, dysphagia, and dysarthria occurred. A repeat CT scan at New York Hospital disclosed a brain stem mass with an enhancing ring and necrotic center (Fig. 1). Surgery revealed a vascular tumor fungating into the cisterns around the obex that proved to be a malignant astrocytoma. Despite radiation therapy and chemotherapy, the child deteriorated progressively and died 4 months later. Autopsy revealed that the tumor had spread along the subarachnoid space to involve the entire neuraxis.

Case 2. The differential diagnosis in the case of H. S. was between a brain stem glioma and a brain stem hemorrhage. Two years before diagnosis, this 23-year-old nurse developed a sudden headache, nausea, vomiting, and left hemiparesis. CT scan and angiogram were normal, and she was told that she probably had an

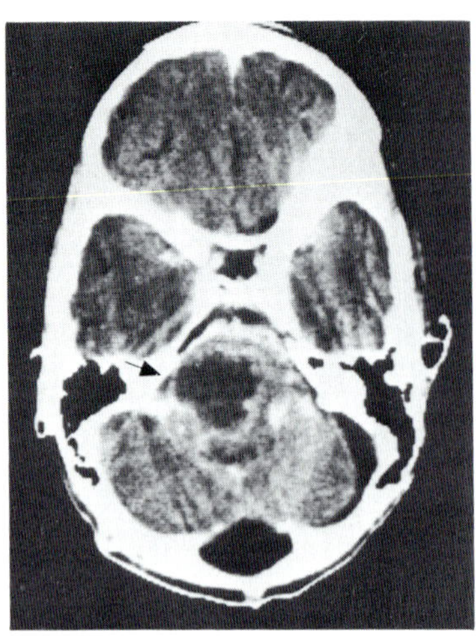

FIG. 1. Malignant brainstem tumor in S. B., a 9-year-old child.

arteriovenous malformation. One year later, the CT scan was repeated and was again normal.

Except for mild left hemiparesis, she did well until 2 months prior to admission when severe headaches, vertigo, nausea, vomiting, and numbness on both sides of the face developed. These improved, but numbness in the left lower and upper limb persisted. CT revealed a lesion in the pons, and the radiologists favored a diagnosis of glioma.

At surgery, the brain stem just beneath the entry zone of the fifth nerve was yellowed and enlarged. An incision was made in the brain stem, and a hematoma was evacuated. Biopsy of the hematoma wall revealed only hemosiderin-laden macrophages. Repeat angiography was normal.

Postoperatively, the patient's gait returned to normal, the numbness on the right side of the body disappeared, and she has resumed her nursing career.

Case 3. The last case was that of a child who was thought to have a brain stem glioma, but because slight fever was present the diagnosis of a brain stem abscess was entertained. Surgery proved this to be the case and a cure was possible.

This 2½-year-old girl had a 3 month history of ataxia, lethargy, slurred speech, vomiting, and drooling. In addition, a low-grade fever was present. Physical examination demonstrated a right hemiparesis, a left sixth nerve palsy, and a tendency to deviate both eyes to the right. The CSF contained three white cells, a glucose of 79 mg%, and a protein of 204 mg%. A CT scan revealed an enhancing mass in the brain stem with a lucid center (Fig. 2). Surgical exploration showed a discoloration of the floor of the fourth ventricle 2 mm caudal to the facial colliculus; 1.5 cc of pus were aspirated and frozen, and pathological section revealed necrotic debris with multiple polymorphonuclear cells. Cultures were positive for *Staphylococcus* and *Streptococcus*. She was treated with antimicrobial therapy and made a complete recovery except for a persistent facial palsy (9).

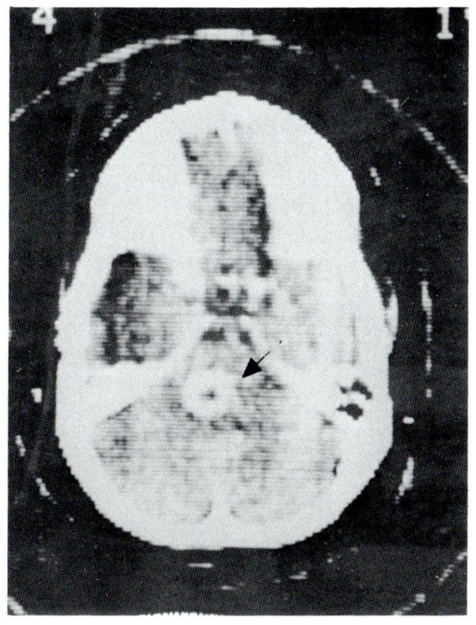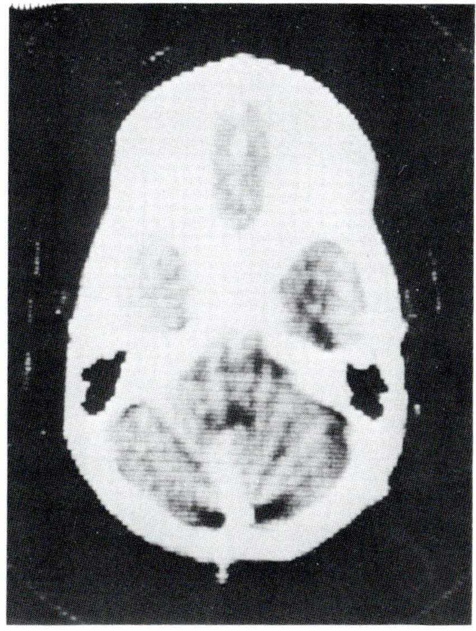

FIG. 2. Left: Brainstem mass in patient V. W. with ring enhancement that proved to be an abscess. **Right:** Enhanced scan after surgery and antimicrobial therapy.

TABLE 1. *Markers in pineal neoplasms*

Tumor	Tumor marker
Embryonal carcinoma	AFP and HCG
Choriocarcinoma	HCG
Endodermal sinus tumor	AFP
Germinoma and teratoma	Neither

AFP = alphafetoprotein, HCG = human chorionic gonadotropin

TUMORS OF THE PINEAL REGION

As a first step in managing tumors of the pineal region, we prefer to obtain blood and spinal fluid for the measurement of alphafetoprotein and human chorionic gonadotropin. If these are positive, then the diagnosis, we believe, is secure, and treatment is begun with either chemotherapy or radiation (1,2). The tumor markers associated with different cell types are listed in Table 1. Should markers be absent, then biopsy is appropriate, as in the following case. D. O., a 26-year-old woman, had a 10-year history of ocular palsy, hydrocephalus, and amenorrhea. Attempted biopsy 6 years earlier was nondiagnostic, and she was treated by a shunting procedure and radiation therapy. Ataxia and paralysis of upper gaze prompted readmission to the hospital, where CT scan revealed a persistent tumor in the region of the pineal gland. A reoperation was performed exposing an infiltrating glioma in the quadrigeminal plate that contained some cystic fluid. Biopsy and partial removal were achieved, and the tissue proved to be astrocytoma. Postoperatively, she was treated with chemotherapy. She returned to work for a time, but increasing neurological deficit then supervened, and she died 2 years later.

The approach that we use to pineal tumors is a hybrid of that popularized by Dr. Bennett Stein and the one favored by Dr. Kemp Clark. It is a supratentorial approach in which the occipital pole is retracted and the tentorium divided near the straight sinus. Instead of dividing the splenium of the corpus callosum and dissecting the great veins, we then divide all the venous connections between the cerebellum and the great veins and follow the route over the cerebellum suggested by Dr. Stein. This provides more room than the suboccipital approach and allows control of the arterial supply from the posterior choroidal arteries (7,11).

TUMORS OF THE LEFT CEREBRAL HEMISPHERE

All tumors of the left hemisphere are approachable, even in the temporal lobe, and in many cases a total excision can be achieved without inducing an unwanted neurological deficit. The case of J. S., who was refused operation in another city, is a good example.

Case 1. J. S., a 66-year-old chief executive officer of a major U.S. corporation, developed difficulty using words 3 months prior to admission. Examination revealed a mild aphasia and a subtle right hemiparesis. CT scan showed a mass in the region of the left trigone, and angiography was normal (Fig. 3).

A craniotomy was performed and an incision 5 cm long was made in the middle temporal gyrus above the ear. At a depth of 4 cm, a tumor was encountered, and a gross total removal was achieved. Postoperatively, the aphasia increased transiently, but by 2 weeks, speech had improved to nearly normal. A postoperative CT scan showed no residual tumor, and he was entered into the brain tumor study group.

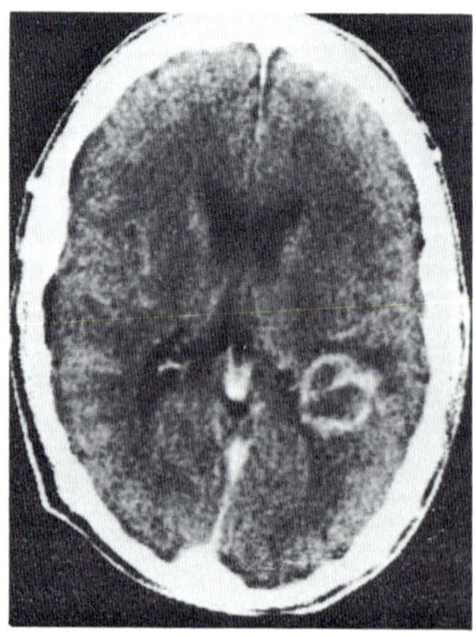

FIG. 3. Left posterior temporal glioma in patient J. S. Gross total excision was achieved without inducing a neurological deficit.

Case 2. As in case 1, patient L. I. had a tumor in the region of the atrium of the left lateral ventricle, which was operated on in a similar fashion. However, the outcome thus far has been better in that the tumor has not recurred.

L. I., a 51-year-old woman, had a history dating back as long as 5 years when she had developed trouble with balance for which she compensated by tilting her head to the left when she walked. In recent months the unsteadiness increased, particularly on moving buses. At times she appeared to have memory lapses, associated with short outbursts of temper and diminished attention span. More recently, headaches developed. Examination revealed mild intellectual impairment and a right homonomous hemianopsia. Dysmetria was present on the right side. CT scan revealed a mass in the region of the atrium of the left lateral ventricle (Fig. 4). A left temporal craniotomy was performed, and a linear incision 6 cm long was made in the middle temporal gyrus above the left ear. At a depth of 2

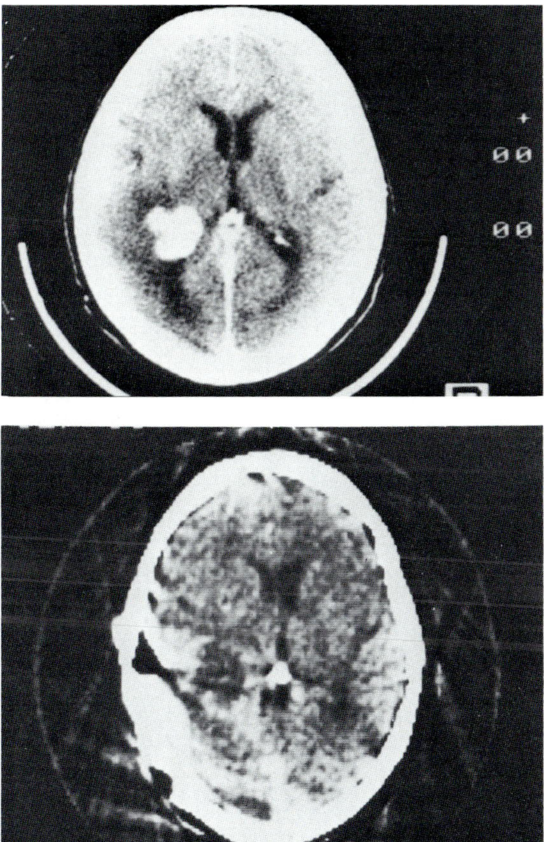

FIG. 4. Top: Left posterior temporal tumor, probably metastatic, in patient L. I. Gross total excision was possible without inducing a neurological deficit. **Bottom:** Postoperative enhanced scan.

cm, a tumor was encountered, and a gross total removal was achieved. Postoperative CT scan revealed no evidence of residual tumor. The pathological diagnosis was unclear, and an extensive search for a primary tumor was negative. One year later she remains well.

The approach to tumors in the region of the atrium is through the middle temporal gyrus above the ear sparing the draining veins of the temporal lobe, as described by Torre et al. (12). Our experience has shown that tumor removal can be accomplished without inducing an important neurological deficit.

TUMORS NEAR THE BASAL GANGLIA

We have observed no serious complications in biopsying tumors of the basal ganglia on either the right or the left side using either stereotaxic or open techniques as illustrated by the following two cases.

Case 1. L. B., an 11-year-old girl, developed ataxia of gait, dysarthria, and a right hemiparesis. CT scan revealed a mass in the region of the left basal ganglia (Fig. 5). In the operating room under anesthesia, air was injected into the lumbar subarachnoid space in the sitting position. The air collected in the frontal horns of the lateral ventricle and in the anterior portion of the third ventricle. A small craniotomy was performed in the left frontal region, and a ventricular needle passed down to the region of the tumor with roentgenographic guidance of the image intensifier. Then a small core of brain was sucked out along the track of the ventricular needle to the region of the tumor, which was generously biopsied. Following operation, her neurological condition did not deteriorate, and she was discharged and given radiation therapy in a total dose of 4,400 rads at the mid-plane.

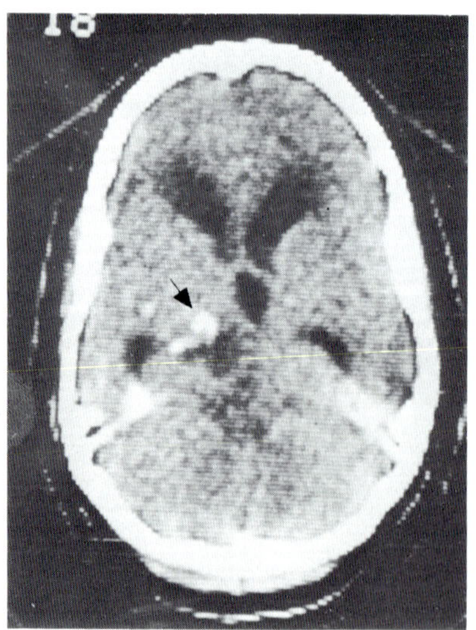

FIG. 5. Deep glioma (patient L. B.) subjected to open biopsy with radiographic control without inducing a neurological deficit.

Six months later, double vision and headaches developed, and CT scan revealed large ventricles, which were corrected by a ventriculo-atrial shunt.

She is now in the tenth grade in school 4½ years after surgery, without palsies, but requiring extra help. Normal menstruation has begun.

Case 2. B. B., a 20-year-old woman, developed a sensation of electric shocks in the left side of her body at age 15. A radioactive brain scan was positive, but the CT scan was not. The seizures were poorly controlled, and she was referred for further management. A CT scan performed at the time of admission revealed a partly calcified mass in the region of the isle of Reil (Fig. 6). The patient was taken to the operating room, and using the image intensifier in the lateral projection, a marker was placed on the scalp overlying the position of the tumor as judged by the radioactive brain scan. A burr hole was made in this region and a blunt needle passed to the appropriate depth under the surface of the brain as judged by the image intensifer. Aspiration biopsies revealed a low-grade, partly calcified astrocytoma. She was treated subsequently by radiation therapy and remains well except for continued difficulty controlling seizures.

A number of authors have described methods of biopsy of tumors using a CT scan. We have employed this in approximately 12 cases and it has proven quite satisfactory—we have experienced no complications. In most cases, a small amount of blood has been identifiable across the course of the needle track, but no symptomatic hemorrhage has ensued (4,5,6,10).

MULTIPLE LESIONS

If multiple lesions are present and no tissue is available, then we prefer to biopsy one of the intracranial lesions. Localization of small lesions can be done in CT scan by a variety of methods that have been amply described in the literature. Sometimes the results are surprising as illustrated by the following cases.

Case 1. Four weeks prior to admission, M. M., a 66-year-old woman, noted numbness and paresthesias which began in the right foot and spread to involve the entire right side of the body. It was followed by difficulty in walking, and CT scan revealed two lesions, one in the region of the left basal ganglia and the second in the left occipital region (Fig. 7). These lesions were thought to be metastatic in origin, and chest X-ray, stool guaiacs, liver function tests, an upper GI series, intravenous pyelogram (IVP), liver scan, and mammography were performed. Mammography demonstrated a 2 cm mass in the breast, but biopsy showed this only to be fibrocystic disease and an intraductal papilloma.

The occipital lesion was localized with the help of computed tomography, and at a depth of 2 cm the tumor was encountered and removed (8). Pathological examination showed the tumor to be a glioblastoma multiforme. She was placed on the protocol of the brain tumor study group.

Case 2. W. M., a 48-year-old woman, presented with a 4-month history of headache, double vision, blurred vision, papilledema, and a mild hemiparesis. CT scan revealed two intracranial lesions, and because no pathological diagnosis was

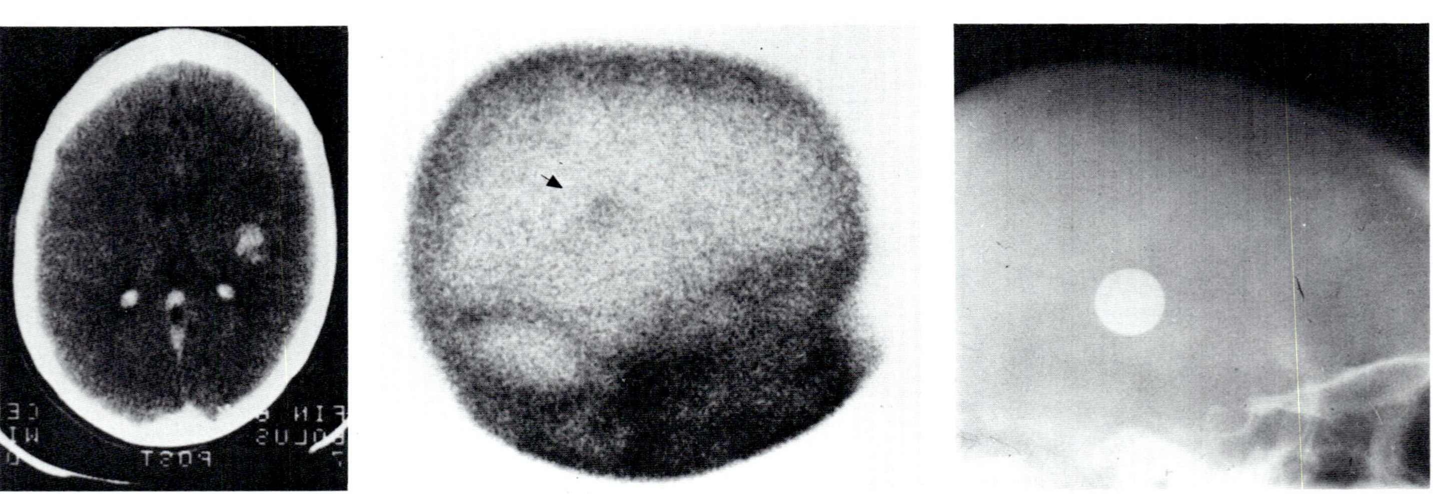

FIG. 6. Centrally placed glioma in the right hemisphere (patient B. B.) which was biopsied with fluoroscopic control in the operating room. **Left:** Enhanced CT scan (patient B.B.) showing the lesion. **Center:** Radionucleotide scan demonstrating the lesion in lateral projection. **Right:** View on image intensifier in which a coin marks the position of the tumor projected on the skull.

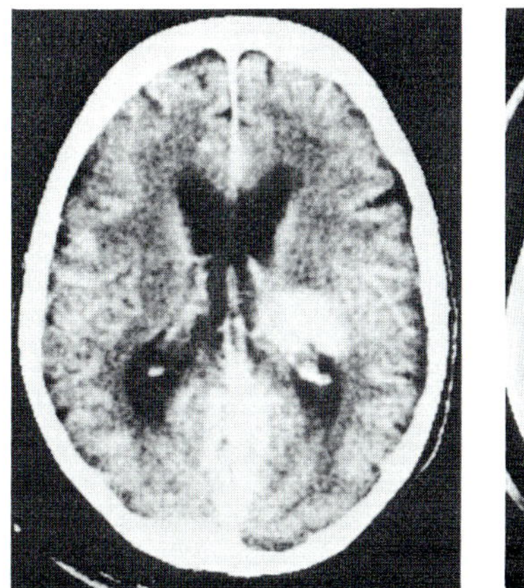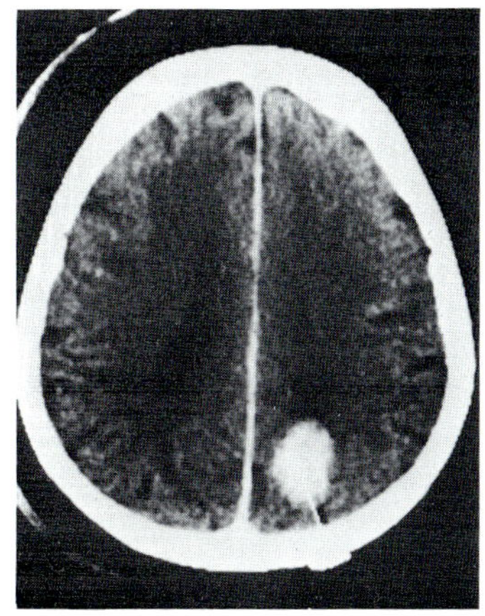

FIG. 7. Patient M. M., initially thought to have multiple metastatic lesions, proved on biopsy to have a glioblastoma multiforme tumor.

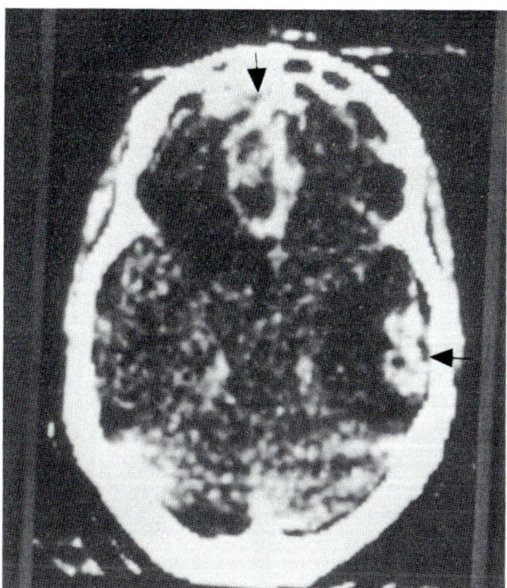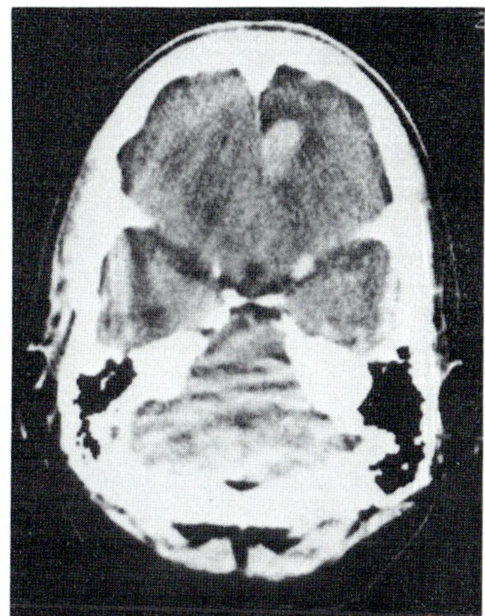

FIG. 8. **Left:** In patient W.M. an enhanced CT scan revealed a left frontal and right parietal enhancing mass. **Right:** CT scan after excision of the right parietal tuberculoma and antimicrobial therapy. A calcified left frontal mass remains.

available, a right parietal craniotomy was performed and one of the lesions was removed (Fig. 8). This proved to be a tuberculoma. This unexpected finding prompted more attention to the patient's past history of a draining axillary sinus. She was treated with antituberculous therapy, and follow-up CT scans revealed a residual area of increased density in the left frontal region, which, however, is asymptomatic.

INTRAVENTRICULAR TUMORS

Intraventricular tumors, as is well known, are quite amenable to surgery. We have used a technique described in the European literature for the biopsy and removal of tumors of the third ventricle that reduces the risk of impairing the short-term memory—the most serious complication of this surgery. If the tumor has destroyed one column of the fornix, then surgical division or injury of the other column of the fornix is likely to induce a severe memory deficit. This can be avoided by enlarging the foramen of Monro posteriorly dividing the thalamostriate vein (Fig. 9). This allows rather lengthy exposure of the entire third ventricle after the choroid plexus is elevated, as illustrated in the following case (3).

C. W., a 15-year-old schoolgirl from the Caribbean, was brought to the U.S. with a history of having developed headaches 11 months prior to admission, followed by difficulty walking that caused her to be bedridden for 8 months, and near blindness for 5 months. Examination revealed that the girl was apathetic, drowsy, poorly oriented, and could not sustain a conversation. Optic atrophy was present, and vision was limited to light perception in each eye. Computed tomography demonstrated a large mass involving the lateral and third ventricles. An angiogram suggested that the cerebral veins were more suitable for an operation on the left side, and so a left frontal craniotomy was performed and the left lateral ventricle entered. Using an ultrasonic aspirator, a good portion of the tumor was removed,

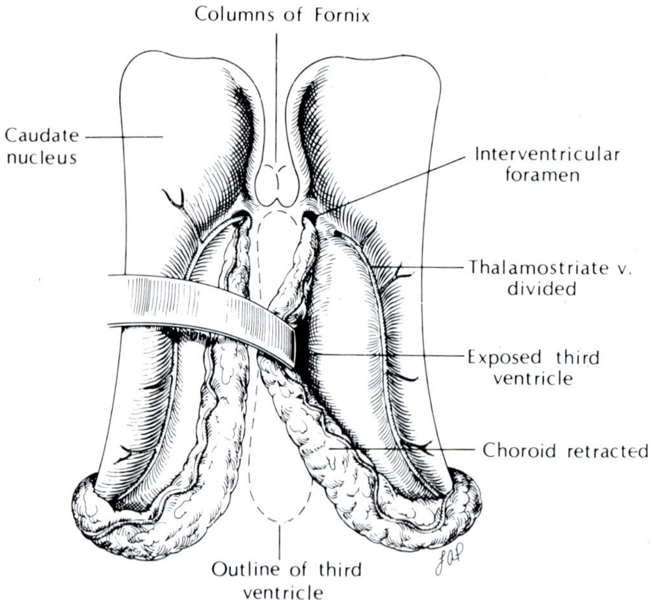

FIG. 9. Maneuver used to open the third ventricle. By incising the foramen of Monro posteriorly, dividing the thalamostriate vein, and cutting the thin attachment of the choroid plexus to the thalamus, the risk of damaging the fornix and impairing memory is reduced.

and a low-pressure ventriculo-atrial shunt was performed at the time of the same operation.

Postoperatively, she remained unimproved. The lateral ventricles did not diminish in size; therefore, 9 days later the low-pressure ventriculo-atrial shunt was converted to an extra low-pressure ventriculo-atrial shunt. Following this procedure, she improved dramatically. She was able to walk by herself, to dress, to eat with table utensils, and to carry on a ready and cheerful conversation. Vision remained unchanged. Pathological examination of the tumor revealed a subependymal giant cell astrocytoma.

One interesting feature of her care was that a low-pressure Holter ventriculo-atrial shunt did not relieve her hydrocephalus; this was only achieved after conversion to an extra low-pressure shunt. At CMC there have been other examples of low-pressure shunts failing to relieve hydrocephalus. Therefore we currently place an extra low-pressure valve in all adults since the syndrome of slit-like ventricles is much less common than in children.

OLD AGE

As the next case illustrates, age per se is not a contraindication to the removal of an intracranial tumor, even if it is suspected of being malignant.

C. G., a 79-year-old woman, was transferred from another hospital with a diagnosis of a right hemispheric stroke. Two and one-half weeks prior to admission she had developed the sudden onset of a left hemiparesis, and a radioactive brain scan was compatible with an infarction in the right cerebral hemisphere. CT scan performed at The New York Hospital was more suggestive of a glioma, measuring approximately 4 cm in diameter. During the examination she was dishevelled and given to sudden outbursts of crying and laughing. She was unable to calculate and could walk only with support.

A right parietal occipital craniotomy was performed, and total removal was achieved judging by the postoperative CT scan. Pathological examination confirmed the clinical impression of glioblastoma multiforme. She tolerated the surgery well, her physical and mental status improved postoperatively, and she became able to walk readily by herself. She was discharged on the 16th postoperative day to the care of a neurologist near her home.

COMMENTS

Virtually all brain tumors can be safely biopsied, with the possible exception of one that produces a smooth and regularly enlarged brain stem that fails to enhance. Most brain stem tumors will have an eccentric mass, well-defined cyst, or an exophytic portion that makes biopsy safe. Hemispheral brain tumors can be operated and very often removed, even from the left hemisphere. An exception to the plan of gross, total removal would be a tumor that extends around major cerebral vessels, such as the middle cerebral trifurcation and the region of the carotid bifurcation. We have found the Cavitron ultrasonic aspirator to be a help because tough, gliotic tumors can be removed without shaking the normal brain. Possibly the carbon dioxide laser will offer similar advantages, but our experience with this is limited. Another technique to increase the safety of removing tumors from near motor or speech areas is to perform the operation under local anesthesia, which permits identifying eloquent areas of the cortex by testing strength and speech or by electrostimulation of the cortex.

Although evidence with both glioma and medulloblastoma suggests that better patient survival is achieved after gross total removal of the tumor, some tumors cannot be totally resected because of their location. Surgical techniques to facilitate the removal of tumors of the pineal region and in the third ventricle are recounted in the text. For deep lesions, one can always resort to aspiration biopsy in the computed tomographic apparatus. The procedure seems safe enough. Often a small amount of blood is seen along the needle track on the post-biopsy computed tomogram, but we have had no worsening of neurological state and no major hemorrhages. Hahn and co-workers reported on 14 cases, and they too reported no complications (4). James et al. (6) had experience with 13 patients, 4 of whom showed increased weakness after freehand needle biopsy of the tumor in the computed tomographic scanning device. All were back to their baseline neurological status within 72 hours. Of 13 patients, 1 showed hemorrhage, but this was asymptomatic.

Some have proposed that it is possible to recognize or distinguish a glioblastoma or a metastasis on the basis of the CT scan alone. Our experience, some of which is recounted above, demonstrates that this is not always the case. Past history and the results of the chest roentgenogram provide a more accurate diagnosis, as was reported by Voorhies et al. (13). They found that in 57 patients with a solitary cerebral tumor and a history of past cancer, 93% had a cerebral metastasis. However, 3 patients had a second primary intracranial neoplasm, and 1 had a non-neoplastic lesion. In the case of 153 patients with a solitary cerebral tumor and no previous diagnosis of cancer, 80% were found to have a primary brain tumor, but 15% had metastatic tumors, and 5% had non-neoplastic lesions. One pertinent question is how much of a preoperative evaluation a patient with a solitary brain tumor should have prior to surgery. According to the authors, the accuracy of the preoperative diagnosis can be increased from the 80% mentioned above to 85% if the chest X-ray is normal. The accuracy goes up to 87% if the patient has a normal chest X-ray and a normal IVP. A further extended work-up is unlikely to reveal a primary tumor in another organ such as the bowel. Consequently, in patients with a solitary tumor and no history of cancer, we favor removal of the tumor if the chest X-ray is normal.

In patients with multiple brain tumors and no histological diagnosis of cancer, biopsy of the brain tumor is also appropriate. Our experience is that this can be safely done. We choose the most superficial tumor and use the computed tomogram to place a marker over the side of the tumor to facilitate the surgery.

Old people, those in their late 70's and 80's, do not tolerate surgery for brain tumor as well as younger patients. However, if the quality of their life does not measure up to their expectations because of a neurological deficit or the effects of edema and pressure from the tumor, then removal of the tumor is reasonable. This presumes that the function of the other vital organs is satisfactory.

REFERENCES

1. Allen, C. F., Nisselbaum, J., Epstein, F., Rosen, G., and Schwartz, M. K. (1979): Alphafetoprotein and human chorionic gonadotropin determination in cerebrospinal fluid. *J. Neurosurg.,* 51:368–374.
2. Arita, N., Bitoh, S., Ushio, Y., Hawakawa, T., Hasegawa, H., Fujiwara, M., Ozaki, K., Parkhen, L., and Mori, T. (1980): Primary pineal endodermal sinus tumor with elevated serum and CSF alphafetoprotein levels. *J. Neurosurg.,* 53:244–248.
3. Delandsheer, J. M., Guyot, J. F., Scherpereel, B., and Laine, E. (1978): Accèss au Troisième Ventricule Par Voi Inter-thalomo-trigonale. *Neurochirurgie,* 24:419–422.
4. Hahn, J. F., Levy, W. J., and Weinstein, M. J. (1979): Needle biopsy of intracranial lesions guided by computerized tomography. *Neurosurgery,* 5:11–15.
5. Jacques, S., Shelden, C. H., McCann, G. D., Freshwater, D. B., and Rand, R. (1980): Computerized three-dimensional stereotaxic removal of small central nervous system lesions in patients. *J. Neurosurg.,* 53:816–820.
6. James, H. E., Wells, M., Alksne, J. F., Wickbom, I., Siemers, P., Brahme, F., and Rosenberg, J. (1979): Needle biopsy under computerized tomographic control: A method for tissue diagnosis in intracranial lesions. *Neurosurgery,* 5:671–674.
7. Lazar, M. L., and Clark, K. (1974): Direct surgical management of masses in the region of the vein of Galen. *Surg. Neurol.,* 2:17–21.
8. King, J. S., and Walker, J. (1980): Precise preoperative localization of intracranial mass lesions. *Neurosurgery,* 6:160–163.
9. Messina, A. V., Guido, L. J., and Liebeskind, A. L. (1977): Preoperative diagnosis of brain stem abscess by computerized tomography with survival. Case report. *J. Neurosurg.,* 47:106–108.
10. Piskun, W. S., Stevens, E. A., Lamorgese, J. R., Paullus, W. S., and Myers, P. W. (1979): A simplified method of CT assisted localization and biopsy of intracranial lesions. *Surg. Neurol.,* 11:413–417.
11. Stein, B. M. (1971): The infratentorial supracerebellar approach to pineal lesions. *J. Neurosurg.,* 35:197–202.
12. Torre, E. D. L., Alexander, E., Jr., Davis, C. H., Jr., and Crandall, D. L. (1963): Tumors of the lateral ventricles of the brain. Report of eight cases, with suggestions for clinical management. *J. Neurosurg.,* 20:461–470.
13. Voorhies, R. M., Sundaresan, N., and Thaler, H. T. (1980): The single supratentorial lesion. An evaluation of preoperative diagnostic tests. *J. Neurosurg.,* 53:364–368.

Controversies in Neurology, edited by R. A.
Thompson and J. R. Green. Raven Press,
New York © 1983.

Asymptomatic Carotid Bruit

Robert M. Crowell*, Robert J. Ojemann**, and J. Philip Kistler**

*Barrow Neurological Institute of St. Joseph's Hospital and Medical Center,
Phoenix, Arizona 85013, and **Massachusetts General Hospital,
Harvard Medical School, Boston, Massachusetts 02114*

With heightened awareness of cerebrovascular disease, physicians often discover asymptomatic carotid bruit during routine physical examinations. Such bruits reflect turbulent blood flow in the internal carotid artery (ICA) due to local atherosclerosis with stenosis. There is evidence that such stenosis may be progressive, eventually leading to hemodynamic insufficiency or distal embolization (4,26). Such events may cause transient ischemic attacks (TIAs) or ischemic infarction. Various strategies have been devised for evaluating and managing patients with asymptomatic carotid bruits. Some physicians have advised careful follow-up (24), while others have proposed antiplatelet therapy (5) or carotid endarterectomy (18,44,45).

The overall management of this condition remains controversial. Unfortunately, satisfactory data are lacking for the natural history of patients with asymptomatic carotid bruits. Since various management protocols have been applied to selected patients, results cannot be reliably compared. Recent work has focused on the role of noninvasive diagnostic tests to guide the management for asymptomatic cervical bruit (1,2,41).

These tests, and the newly developed method of digital subtraction angiography (9), lend themselves to minimal risk characterization of the pathologic anatomy in populations of patients. Studies of other cerebrovascular problems have familiarized clinical neuroscientists with the powerful techniques of epidemiology and randomized clinical trials (5). Appropriate studies must be mounted to provide the control data necessary to settle the question of optimum management in these patients.

ETIOLOGY

Cervical bruits may arise from a variety of pathologic conditions (Table 1) (18). Internal carotid artery stenosis is probably the commonest and certainly the most important condition giving rise to cervical bruit. Other conditions which sometimes cause neck bruits are carotid dissection, external carotid artery stenosis, transmitted bruits from the great vessels of the thorax, and radiated cardiac murmurs. Unusual causes of cervical bruit include venous hum, internal carotid artery kink, and fibromuscular dysplasia (18).

TABLE 1. *Differential diagnosis of cervical bruit*

Internal carotid artery stenosis
External carotid artery stenosis
Internal carotid artery dissection
Internal carotid artery kink
Fibromuscular dysphasia
Subclavian artery stenosis
Radiated cardiac murmur
High output state (hyperthyroidism)
Intracranial arteriovenous malformation
Carotid cavernous fistula
Venous hum

The pathologic process underlying the usual ICA stenosis is atherosclerosis which does not differ importantly from the form of atherosclerosis which commonly affects the coronary and peripheral arteries. Atheroma tends to accumulate in the posterior aspect of the distal, common, and proximal interal carotid arteries, and to a lesser extent in the proximal external carotid artery. For a bruit to occur, there must be more than 70% reduction in the cross-sectional area of the arterial lumen; the lumen diameter must therefore be reduced more than 50% (21). Because of the difficulty of estimating percentage diameter reduction from angiography, it is more practical and reliable to estimate residual lumen diameter in millimeters. Bruits generally occur when the residual lumen diameter is 3 mm or less (30). Bruits are produced by turbulent jets of blood just distal to the stenosis. This turbulent flow is related to the residual flow rate in the poststenotic segment which in turn is related to the residual lumen diameter at the stenosis. The higher the pitch of a bruit, the tighter the stenosis. High-pitched bruits extending into diastole are of particular importance because of their close association to tightly stenotic lesions with residual lumen diameter less than 2 mm. When stenosis reaches this extent, reduction of distal flow can be expected. Collateral circulation through the circle of Willis tends to maintain pressure in the intracranial carotid artery. When residual lumen diameter falls below 1 mm, with impending occlusion, the bruit diminishes in intensity (30). With ICA occlusion, the bruit may disappear.

The pathophysiology of cerebral and retinal symptoms above a bruit producing stenotic lesion is unsettled (Fig. 1). Fisher brought attention to the relationship between carotid occlusive disease and stroke (19,20), and it was thought for some time that the major mechanism of stroke was occlusion with inadequate distal cerebral perfusion (19). More recently, attention has focused on embolization from the carotid bifurcation to intracranial vessels as a mechanism of stroke (3,34,38). Embolization may occur from stenosis, thrombosis, or ulceration at the carotid bifurcation. The asymptomatic carotid bruit might therefore act as a harbinger of disastrous stroke emanating from stenosis or eventual thrombosis. Recently, careful studies have indicated that tight ICA stenosis often leads to TIA (37). Epidemiologic data have indicated that TIA is followed by stroke occurring at a rate of about 5 per year (47). More recent investigations, supported with careful angiography and

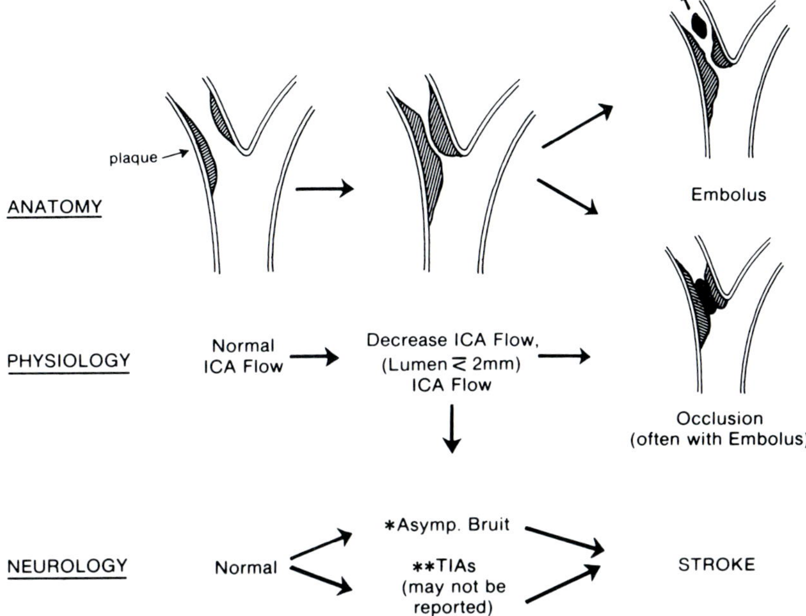

FIG. 1. Pathophysiology of carotid occlusive disease.

CT data, indicate that this stroke rate after TIA depends heavily on the specific pathologic anatomy leading to TIA (3,34). There is some evidence that the tight ICA stenosis (less than 2-mm residual lumen) leads to a high frequency of cerebral infarction, but further careful angiographic-clinical correlation will be needed to confirm this point.

NATURAL HISTORY

The pathologic anatomy associated with cervical bruit is highly variable. Cervical bruits can be generated by variable degrees of stenosis in the ICA. Stenosis may or may not be associated with ulceration, and atherosclerotic lesions progress at varying rates. The natural history of these conditions is as variable as the underlying anatomic configurations.

Efforts to define the natural history of asymptomatic carotid bruit have been restricted by inherent selection factors. Angiographic criteria have the advantage of precision in anatomic diagnosis but are by their very nature highly selected. Series based on criteria developed by noninvasive diagnostic techniques are significantly less precise in anatomic diagnosis though broader populations of patients may be surveyed. Epidemiologic studies may be population-based and prospective in their data-gathering; however, such investigations generally rely on auscultation for a diagnosis, and the anatomic precision is less satisfactory. Given the restrictions of these various types of data, it is not surprising that conflicting data are reported (Table 2).

TABLE 2. *Risk of stroke in patients with carotid bruit/stenosis*

Subjects	Test/criterion	% strokes per year	Reference
Population	Auscultation	0.2%	Wolf et al. (48)
Population	Auscultation	0.7%	Heyman et al. (23)
2nd side[a]	Angiography/50% stenosis	0.9%	Humphries et al. (24)
2nd side[a]	Angiography/50% stenosis	1.7%	Levin and Sondheimer (32)
Selected	Angiography/50% stenosis	4.5%	Thompson (46)

[a]Asymptomatic carotid studied at the time of angiographic study of a contralateral symptomatic carotid lesion.

A number of reports suggest that the natural history of asymptomatic bruit is relatively benign. Humphries et al. (24) reported a series of 168 patients with angiographically demonstrable carotid stenosis of greater than 50% with an average follow-up of 32 months. Twenty-six of this group of patients developed TIAs, and therefore underwent endarterectomy, while 4 patients developed frank stroke—one of these without prior TIAs. If stricter criteria of carotid stenosis had been employed, for example a residual lumen diameter of 2 mm or less, the rate of TIA and stroke might well have been higher. Epidemiologic studies have also suggested a low stroke rate for asymptomatic carotid bruit. Kagan (28) reported a stroke rate of 1% per year, and strokes were regarded as "mild" in a population of Oriental extraction. Wolf et al. (48) investigated in prospective fashion asymptomatic bruits in a large population of patients in Framingham, Massachusetts. Among 245 patients, 5 developed strokes relevant to the apparent carotid stenosis over a period of 12 years for a stroke rate of 0.16% per year. Multiple examiners documented these bruits, and the precise characteristics of the bruits were not specified. Heyman et al. (23) reported on a series of 72 patients followed for an average of 6 years. Three strokes clearly relevant to the bruit in question were recorded for a stroke rate of 0.7% per year. In this study, one single observer recorded the various bruits, the specific characteristics of which were clearly defined.

Other angiographic and clinical studies have suggested a more serious natural history for patients with asymptomatic bruits. Javid and co-workers (26) performed serial angiograms in patients with asymptomatic bruit with follow-up intervals from 1 to 9 years. They found 51 of 86 cases with significant progression of the asymptomatic angiographic stenosis. Kartchner presented data based on noninvasive diagnostic studies which indicated progression of hemodynamic stenosis in 30 of 1,287 patients (29). In this same series, 13 patients of 78 with hemodynamically significant stenosis developed stroke in a 2-year follow-up for an average of 8.3% strokes per year. Thompson and co-workers followed 138 patients with asymptomatic carotid stenosis demonstrated angiographically. These patients were not operated on for a variety of clinical reasons. Twenty-four developed stroke over an average follow-up of 46 months for an average of 4.5% strokes per year (44). This series, which reports a very high stroke rate for asymptomatic stenosis, is complicated by the multiplicity of factors utilized in selecting this group, for example significant medical risk factors, patient preference for medical therapy, etc.

Sources of clinical data other than follow-up of asymptomatic bruit have provided indirect evidence that this condition may lead suddenly to unacceptable neurological deficit. C. M. Fisher studied 50 cases of interal carotid occlusion (19). Among these patients, 8 cases (16%) were asymptomatic and 13 (26%) experienced TIA or mild stroke with good recovery. By contrast, however, 29 cases (58%) suffered moderate to severe neurological deficit considered an unacceptable result. In the cases of frank stroke, 60% had prior TIAs but 40% experienced no warning attacks of any sort. Similar findings were found by Pessin et al. (38), wherein 64 patients with acute carotid stroke had documentation of previous TIAs in 54% but no warning in 46%.

Presently, there is no way to predict in a given asymptomatic patient what the outcome will be. Awaiting the occurrence of warning TIAs to identify the patients at risk means settling for a potentially unacceptable outcome in approximately 30% of the cases. These data support the position that management of asymptomatic carotid occlusive disease may be critical in reducing the incidence of stroke (33). An additional problem arises from the unreliability of patients, even the most sophisticated, in reporting TIAs, despite extensive discussion of TIAs and their significance.

An additional condition related to the asymptomatic bruit is the asymptomatic ICA ulcer. These lesions have commonly been regarded as benign, but Moore et al. have recently presented evidence to suggest that deep and irregular lesions may cause stroke in as many as 12.5% of cases per year (35).

Another aspect of the asymptomatic carotid stenosis problem is the question of increased risk of stroke in such patients during major surgery, such as cardiac or peripheral-vascular for example. Fields (18) and other workers have reported an incidence of stroke of 3 to 5% in this type of patient. A host of recent studies, based on auscultation and noninvasive diagnostic data, have indicated a very low rate of perioperative stroke in these patients (6,8,17,46). On the other hand, Kartchner found that patients with hemodynamically significant stenosis or occlusion on noninvasive investigation have a substantial rate of stroke during cardiac surgery (29).

EVALUATION

Bedside clinical examination can assist in the characterization of the pathologic anatomy at the carotid bifurcation (Fig. 2). Most internal carotid stenoses are associated with bruits which are localized to the midcervical region; that is, these bruits are not heard in the low neck or chest. Moreover a high-pitched bruit suggests a tight carotid stenosis. David and co-workers (12) reported that high-pitched bruits were associated with angiographic narrowing of 50% or more in 95% of their cases. Bruits which are prolonged into diastole are particularly suggestive of marked stenosis as demonstrated angiographically (7,30). A technique of dynamic palpation

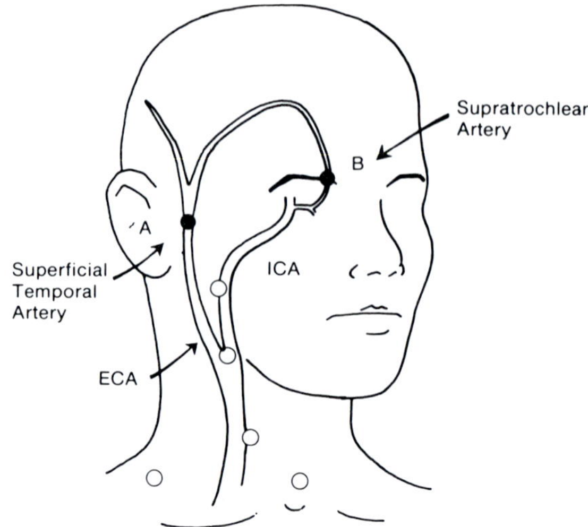

○ Points for auscultation for bruit and palpation for thrill

● Pulses for dynamic palpation test. Compress A, if B is obliterated
then ICA obstruction is suggested.

FIG. 2.   Signs of carotid occlusive disease.

of the facial pulses as described by Ackerman (1,2) can also be useful, when reliable endpoints can be obtained, in the bedside diagnosis of hemodynamically significant carotid occlusive disease. Determination of central retinal artery pressures by ophthalmodynamometry (ODN) is said to provide reliable evidence of significant hemodynamic internal carotid or ophthalmic occlusive disease with approximately 90% accuracy.

A host of techniques for noninvasive diagnosis have been devised to assess carotid occlusive disease (Table 3). The characteristic pitfalls and utilization of these techniques have been discussed in detail (1,10,22,29,41). In general, it may be said that such tests can identify hemodynamically significant ICA stenosis with an accuracy of 85 to 90%. The reliability of the determinations seems to be improved when a battery of tests is employed. Kartchner has indicated that the combination of oculoplethymography (OPG) and direct bruit analysis provides accurate diagnosis of significant hemodynamic carotid stenosis in 89.5% of the cases (29). Experienced clinicians have found these methods particularly reliable in ruling *in* arteriography in a variety of borderline clinical settings including elderly patients with uncertain history for TIA, cases with relative medical contraindications to angiography, and patients with a good recovery from carotid territory cerebral infarction. It has been emphasized that noninvasive diagnostic techniques are not a substitute for standard angiography which is used as the final arbiter of hemodynamically significant carotid stenosis.

TABLE 3. *Noninvasive tests for carotid occlusive disease*

I. Indirect-Orbital circulation
    A. Superficial
        Dymanic palpation of pulses
        Thermography
        Doppler ultrasonography[a]
    B. Deep
        Ophthalmodynamometry (ODN)
        Oculoplethymography (OPG)
        Oculotonography
II. Direct
    Bruit analysis
    Phonogiography[a] (Spectra view)
    Doppler imaging (Echoflow)
    B scan imaging[a]

[a]Combination provides 85–90% accuracy in detection of hemodynamically significant occlusive lesions.

Our own experience demonstrates that a combination of orbital Doppler studies of collateral circulation and quantitative phonoangiography (13) has reliably identified hemodynamically significant carotid stenosis (Fig. 3). Quantitative phonoangiography (13,30) analyzes the frequency-intensity sound spectrum of the carotid bruit and accurately estimates the residual lumen diameter at the point of stenosis. Additionally, this test differentiates between bruits arising at the carotid bifurcation and those emanating from the thorax. Another test which may be helpful is B-scan ultrasonography (10). This technique can beautifully image carotid stenosis in some cases, but in some instances the images have provided disappointing resolution.

Angiography remains the most reliable method for characterizing internal carotid artery stenosis (Fig. 4). In addition to accurately assessing the presence and degree of proximal internal carotid stenosis, angiography reveals the status of intracranial arteries, collateral circulation, and ulcerated plaques. At the moment, carotid angiography is the only technique which can reliably pinpoint carotid artery pathology which is likely to lead to cerebral infarction. As a prelude to carotid endarterectomy, we recommend at least bilateral carotid studies. The major drawback to cerebral angiography is the significant risk of lasting neurologic complication.

Computed tomography may be of use in some cases of asymptomatic bruit. In patients with vague symptomatology, CT may demonstrate silent cerebral infarction. The presence of such lesions may, in some instances, indicate that the asymptomatic carotid stenosis has produced cerebral pathology without apparent clinical symptomatology.

Digital subtraction angiography is an exciting new prospect for the low-risk investigation of cerebral vascular disease including asymptomatic carotid bruit (Fig. 5) (9). Briefly, this technique utilizes an intravenous injection of contrast material; the carotid bifurcation is visualized with fluoroscopy and computerized enhancement of the resulting image. The technique at present provides visualization of the carotid bifurcation with resolution only slightly less satisfactory than standard intra-arterial

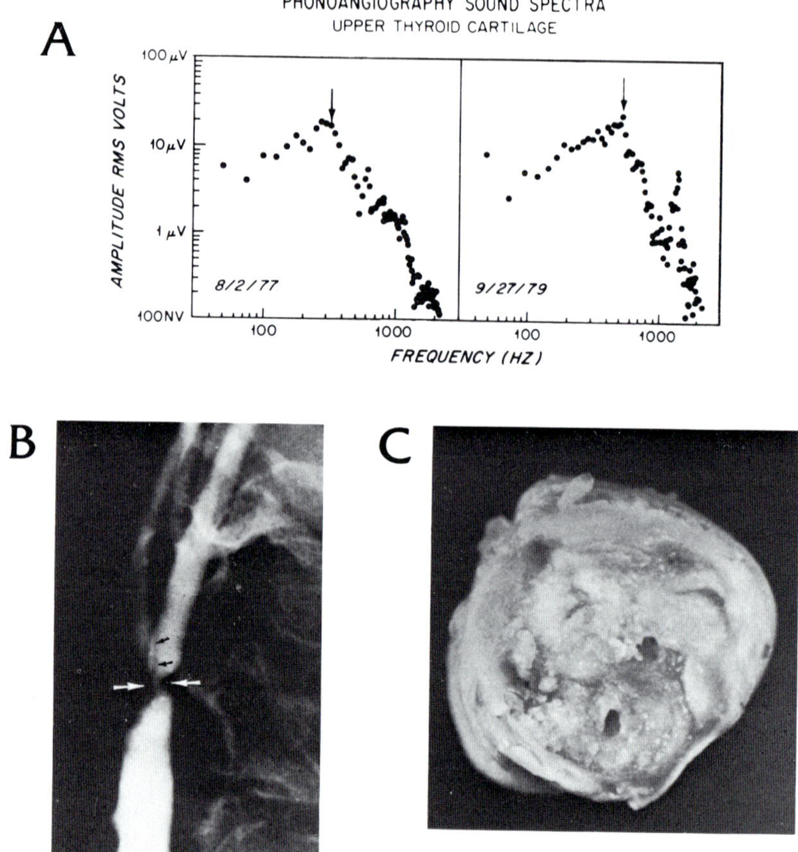

FIG. 3. Management of asymptomatic carotid bruit. **A:** Phonoangiography documents increasing bruit frequency suggesting decreasing residual lumen to under 2 mm. **B:** Angiography confirms residual lumen less than 2 mm *(white arrows)*. **C:** Surgical specimen (cross-section) shows only a pinhole residual lumen. Smooth postoperative course.

carotid angiography. The presence and extent of carotid stenosis may be estimated along with visualization of carotid ulceration and intracranial collateral circulation. Special problems arise from the simultaneous opacification of all the great vessels in the neck. Improved resolution is likely in view of the substantial research and industrial effort in this area at present. Digital subtraction angiography is likely to provide, with minimal risk, quantitative anatomic data on ICA stenosis in patients with asymptomatic carotid bruit.

MANAGEMENT

Reliable guidelines for the management of the asymptomatic carotid bruit have not been established. Consequently, controversies exist regarding the value of antiplatelet or anticoagulant pharmacotherapy, and the indications for carotid endar-

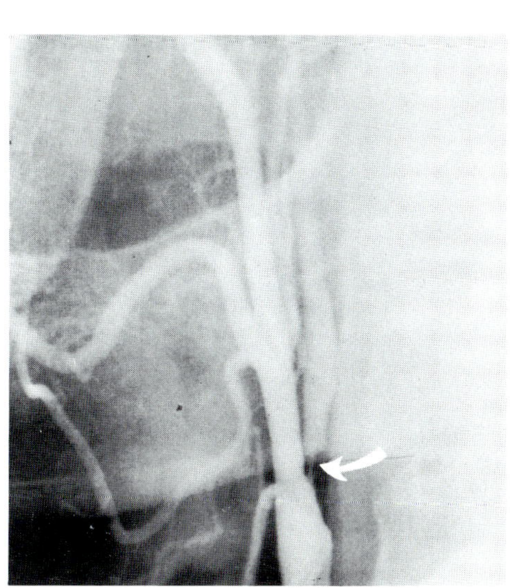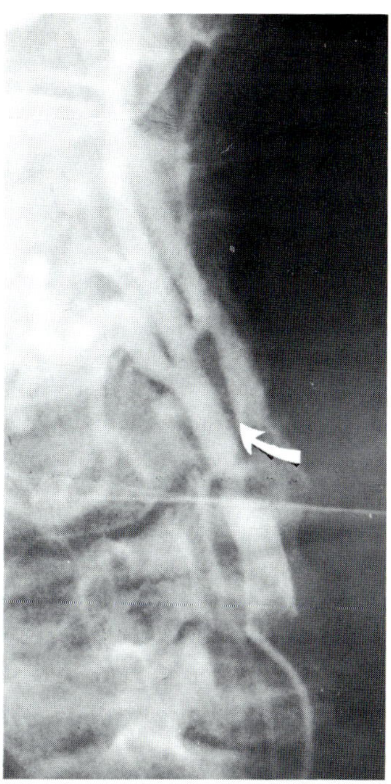

FIG. 4. Asymptomatic left carotid stenosis discovered during evaluation of right-sided symptomatic lesion. Left carotid angiogram shows marked stenosis with residual lumen less than 1.5 mm. Ten days after right carotid endarterectomy, left carotid endarterectomy was performed uneventfully. Patient was heparinized between procedures.

terectomy. Evidence has been presented that antiplatelet therapy for patients with TIAs may diminish the subsequent frequency of stroke, at least for males (5). No evidence has been adduced with regard to the impact of antiplatelet therapy on the eventual stroke rate in patients with asymptomatic bruit (18). Anticoagulation with sodium warfarin, Coumadin®, has long been utilized to ward off stroke, but its efficacy in patients with TIAs has not been proved (4). The advantage of sodium warfarin for patients with asymptomatic bruit has not been established, and many physicians would be hesitant to prescribe this drug which has significant complications.

Several authors have recommended carotid endarterectomy for patients with asymptomatic bruit (26,32,43,45,46). It must be pointed out that satisfactory evidence has not been presented to date that carotid endarterectomy improves the eventual outcome even for patients with TIAs, much less for patients with asymptomatic lesions (4). When considering a surgical therapy, it is important to note complications of the surgical procedure itself (Table 4). It is demonstrated that in several series of elective carotid endarterectomy, complication rates varied dramatically, from 1% in experienced hands (33,36,42,43) to 21% in a community hospital setting (16). Haas has suggested that for elective carotid endarterectomy

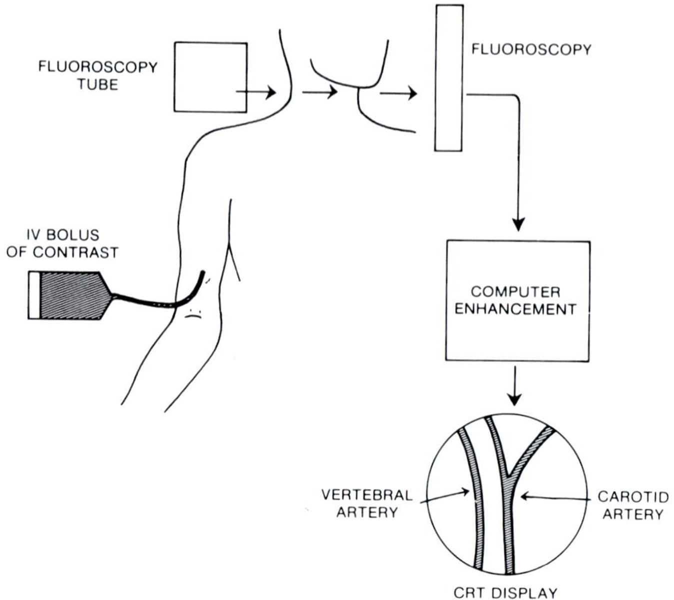

FIG. 5.   Digital subtraction angiography.

TABLE 4. *Risk of carotid endarterectomy for asymptomatic stenosis (or ulceration)*

No. of patients	Stroke	Death	Total risk	Reference
167	2	0	1.2%	Thompson, et al., 1976 (43).
78	0	0	0	Moore, et al., 1979 (35).
30	0	0	0	Crowell, et al., 1981 (11).

for TIA, an operative risk of 2.9% or less should be demonstrated in order to justify the advantage of surgical therapy (27). Sundt has reported that the complication rate is dependent on the preoperative condition of the patient; for neurologically and medically stable patients his complication rate is 1%, whereas the same operator experiences 8% complications in medically and neurologically unstable patients (42). Similarly, Thompson has reported two strokes in 167 operations for asymptomatic carotid bruit (1.2%), and Moore has reported no complications in 78 operations per asymptomatic carotid ulcer (35). In our own clinic, no complications were noted in 30 operations for asymptomatic carotid stenosis (11). Fields has suggested that endarterectomy can be recommended for asymptomatic carotid stenosis only if the complication rate is less than 1% (18). Several authors have emphasized that the complication rate can be minimized when the operator is experienced, carries out the procedure frequently, and utilizes a standard and meticulous technique (40,41). We have described the technique we prefer for carotid endarterectomy (37). Additionally, careful perioperative medical management, particularly in regard to the cardiac status and control of hypertension, is indicated to minimize risk (14,36,39,42).

Other authors, notably Humphries (24), have suggested that patients with asymptomatic carotid stenosis be followed until the appearance of TIAs, at which time surgery is recommended since the risk of cerebral infarction is then greater than the risk of operation (Fig. 6).

The effect of carotid endarterectomy on late stroke occurrence has been assessed in patients presenting with TIAs (49). The incidence of late stroke after carotid endarterectomy was low (Table 2) in Thompson's patients with asymptomatic carotid stenosis; 6 of 132 patients experienced stroke in an average of 55 months follow-up for an average stroke rate of 0.99% per year (44).

DISCUSSION

It is clear from the foregoing discussion that more data is needed to establish optimum management for the patient with asymptomatic carotid bruit. It is known that the best scientific method for establishing a treatment regimen is the randomized

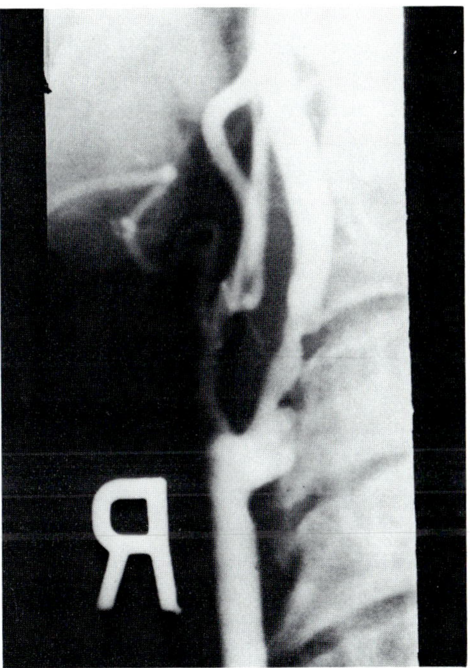

FIG. 6. Known internal carotid stenosis followed until TIA. This 48-year-old woman had a left carotid endarterectomy for ulcerated stenosing plaque with TIAs. Right carotid angiography seen here showed a moderate right internal stenosis which was managed with ASA and observation. After the occurrence of right amaurosis fugax, right endarterectomy was carried out without complication.

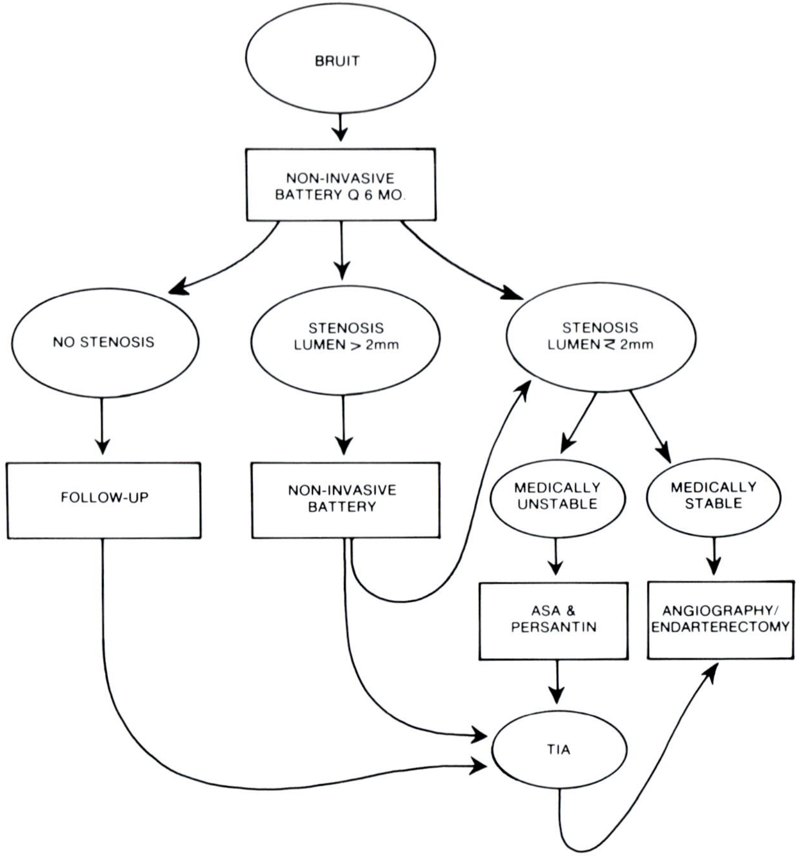

FIG. 7. Diagram for management of asymptomatic carotid bruit.

controlled clinical trial. An ethical study for asymptomatic bruit would likely compare the impact of antiplatelet therapy and carotid endarterectomy. Crossovers to surgical therapy resulting from the occurrence of TIAs would likely drive up the sample size to impractical levels; one estimate of 1,500 has been recently developed (G. G. Ferguson, *personal communication*). If this optimum sort of controlled study is not feasible, the next best tactic might be a registry of cases undergoing various forms of therapy, but all carefully characterized with regard to pathologic anatomy either by cerebral angiography or digital subtraction angiography. This method of study, though less satisfying from the statistician's standpoint, might provide useful data on the natural history of various subsets of asymptomatic carotid stenosis. Certainly additional data regarding natural history would be of great value in guiding management of these cases. The existence of digitized subtraction angiography is very likely to increase the numbers of such patients which confront the neurologic physician and surgeon in the future.

Some reports have recommended surgery for patients with asymptomatic bruit (26,43,45,46). This literature has indicated a high risk of stroke in these patients, a low risk of carotid endarterectomy, and thus a benefit from surgery. Data indicating low risk of stroke from asymptomatic stenosis (23,24,48) and data indicating a high risk of carotid endarterectomy in some hands (16) have cast some doubts on the widespread use of surgery for this condition (4). Humphries recommended surgery when TIAs develop (24). Others have suggested that patients with asymptomatic bruit be given antiplatelet therapy to prevent TIAs and stroke (15), but firm data to support this contention are lacking.

We take the view that certain bruits, those associated with lumen diameter of less than 2 mm, place the patient at greater risk of TIA and stroke. Clinical examination and some noninvasive techniques (phonoangiography) permit the physician to follow patients with asymptomatic bruit to determine when hemodynamically significant stenosis has developed. Only when stenosis of this severity is demonstrated do we seriously consider angiography and subsequent surgery (Fig. 7). When the patient is young and demonstrates bilateral stenosis, the inclination to operate is greater. In older patients, especially those with significant medical risk, antiplatelet therapy can be recommended, as is currently the widespread practice. Following this program, we have operated upon 30 patients with asymptomatic carotid stenosis without any operative morbidity or mortality. A few of these cases demonstrated progressive stenosis on serial study, and all cases had carotid stenosis of 2 mm or less in angiography. We have not been impressed that patients with carotid bruit associated with residual lumen diameter greater than 2 mm run a greater risk of stroke from major surgery, and therefore we have not offered endarterectomy to this category of patient.

REFERENCES

1. Ackerman, R. H. (1980): Non-invasive diagnosis of carotid disease. Cerebrovascular Survey Report, NINCDS.
2. Ackerman, R. H. (1976): The relative effectiveness of six non-invasive tests for carotid disease. *Neurology (Minneap.)*, 26:379–380.
3. Barnett, H. J. M. (1980a): The pathophysiology of transient cerebral ischemic attacks. *Med. Clin. North Am.*, 64:640–675.
4. Barnett, H. J. M. (1980b): Progress towards stroke prevention. *Neurology*, 30:1212–1225.
5. Barnett, H. J. M. et al. (1978): A randomized trial of aspirin and sulfinpyrazone in threatened stroke. The Canadian Cooperative Study Group. *N. Engl. J. Med.*, 299:53.
6. Berkoff, H., and Turnipseed, W. (1979): Postsurgical stroke in cardiac and peripheral vascular disease. *Stroke*, 10:106.
7. Bone, G. E., and Barnes, R. W. (1976): Limitations of the Doppler cerebrovascular examination in hemispheric cerebral ischemia. *Surgery*, 79:577.
8. Carney, W. I., Steward, W. B., DePinto, D. J., et al. (1977): Carotid bruit as a risk in aortoiliac reconstruction. *Surgery*, 81:567.
9. Christensen, P. C., Ovitt, T. W., Fisher, D., et al. (1979): Intravenous cervical carotid angiography utilizing digital video subtraction system. *Proceedings of the 17th Annual Meeting of the American Society of Neuroradiology*, Toronto.
10. Cooperberg, P. L., Robertson, W. D., Fry, P., et al. (1979): High-resolution real-time ultrasound of the carotid bifurcation. *J. Clin. Ultrasound*, 7:13–17.

11. Crowell, R. M., and Ojemann, R. G. (1981): Carotid endarterectomy. In: *Practice of Surgery*, edited by J. T. Hoff. Harper & Row, Hagerstown, Maryland.

12. David, T. E., Humphries, A. W., Young, J. R., and Bevan, E. G. (1973): A correlation of neck bruits and arteriosclerotic carotid arteries. *Arch. Surg.*, 107:729–731.

13. Duncan, G. W., Gruber, J. O., Dewey, C. F., et al. (1975): Evaluation of carotid stenosis by phonoangiography. *N. Engl. J. Med.*, 293:1124.

14. Duncan, G. W., Lees, R. S., Ojemann, R. G., and David, S. S. (1977): Concomitants of atherosclerotic carotid artery stenosis. *Stroke*, 8:665–669.

15. Eastcott, H. H. G., Pickering, G. W., and Rob, C. (1954): Reconstruction of the interal carotid artery in a patient with intermittent attacks of hemiplegia. *Lancet*, 2:994.

16. Easton, J. D., and Sherman, D. G. (1977): Stroke and mortality rate in carotid endarterectomy: 228 consecutive operations. *Stroke*, 8:565–571.

17. Evans, W. E., and Cooperman, M. (1978): The significance of asymptomatic unilateral carotid bruits in preoperative patients. *Surgery*, 83:521.

18. Fields, W. S. (1978): The asymptomatic carotid bruit—Operate or not? *Stroke*, 9:269–271.

19. Fisher, C. M. (1976): The natural history of carotid occlusion. In: *Microneurosurgical Anastomoses for Cerebral Ischemia*, edited by G. M. Austin, pp. 194–201. Charles C. Thomas Publishers, Springfield, Illinois.

20. Fisher, C. M. (1951): Occlusion of the internal carotid artery. *Arch. Neurol. Psychiatry*, 69:346–377.

21. Flanigin, D. P., Tullis, J. P., Streeter, V. L., et al. (1977): Multiple subcritical arterial stenosis—effect on poststenotic pressure and flow. *Ann. Surg.*, 186:663–668.

22. Gee, W., Oller, D. W., and Wylie, E. J. (1976): Non-invasive diagnosis of carotid occlusion by ocular pneumoplethysmography. *Stroke*, 7:18.

23. Heyman, A., Wilkinson, W., Heydon, S., et al. (1980): Risk of stroke in asymptomatic persons with cervical arterial bruits—a population study in Evans County, Georgia. *N. Engl. J. Med.*, 302:838–841.

24. Humphries, A. W., Young, J. R., Santilli, P. H., et al. (1976): Unoperated, asymptomatic significant internal carotid artery stenosis: A review of 182 instances. *Surgery*, 80:695.

25. Javid, H., Ostermiller, W. E., Hengesh, J. W., et al. (1971): Carotid endarterectomy for asymptomatic patients. *Arch. Surg.*, 102:389–391.

26. Javid, H., Ostermiller, W. E., Hengesh, J. W., et al. (1970): Natural history of carotid bifurcation atheroma. *Surgery*, 67:80.

27. Jonas, S., and Haas, W. K. (1979): An approach to the maximal acceptable stroke complication rate after surgery for transient cerebral ischemia. 10:104.

28. Kagan, A., Popner, J., Rhoads, G. G., et al. (1976): Epidemiologic studies on coronary artery disease and stroke in Japanese men living in Japan, Hawaii, and California: Prevalence of stroke. In: *Cerebrovascular Diseases*, edited by P. Scheinberg, pp. 267–277. Raven Press, New York.

29. Kartchner, M. M., and McRae, L. D. (1977): Non-invasive evaluation and management of the "asymptomatic" carotid bruit. *Surgery*, 82:840.

30. Kistler, J. P., Lees, R. S., Friedman, J., et al. (1978): The bruit of carotid stenosis versus radiated basal heart murmurs. Differentiation by phonoangiography. *Circulation*, 57:975–981.

31. Lefrak, E. A., and Guinn, G. A. (1974): Prophylactic carotid artery surgery in patients requiring a second operation. *South Med. J.*, 67:185–189.

32. Levin, S. M., and Sondheimer, F. K. (1976): Stenosis of the contralateral asymptomatic carotid artery—To operate or not? *Vasc. Surg.*, 7:3.

33. Mohr, J. P. (1978): Transient ischemic attacks and the prevention of strokes. *N. Engl. J. Med.*, 299:93–95.

34. Mohr, J. P., Caplan, L. R., Milski, J. M., et al. (1978): The Harvard Cooperative Stroke Registry: A prospective registry of patients hospitalized with stroke. *Neurology (Minneap.)*, 28:754–762.

35. Moore, W. S., Malone, J. M., Boren, C., et al. (1979): Asymptomatic ulcerative lesions of the carotid artery—Natural history and effect of surgical therapy compared. *Stroke*, 10:96.

36. Ojemann, R. G., et al. (1975): Surgical treatment of extracranial carotid occlusive disease. *Clin. Neurosurg.*, 22:214–263.

37. Pessin, M. S., Duncan, G. W., Mohr, J. P., et al. (1977): Clinical and angiographic features of carotid transient ischemic attacks. *N. Engl. J. Med.*, 296:358–362.

38. Pessin, M. S., Hinton, R. C., Davis, K. R., et al. (1979): Mechanisms of acute carotid stroke. *Ann. Neurol.*, 6:245–252.

39. Robertson, J. T. (1976): A neurosurgical approach to the therapy of extracranial occlusive disease. *Clin. Neurosurg.*, 23:1–11.
40. Robertson, J. T., and Watridge, C. B. (1979): The surgical management of extracranial and intracranial occlusive disease. *Med. Clin. North Am.*, 63:681–693.
41. Sandok, B. A. (1978): Non-invasive techniques for diagnosis of carotid artery disease (Editorial). *Stroke*, 9:427.
42. Sundt, T. M., Jr., Sandok, B. A., and Whisnant, J. P. (1975): Carotid endarterectomy: Complications and preoperative assessment of risk. *Mayo Clin. Proc.*, 50:301–306.
43. Thompson, J. E., Austin, D. J., and Patman, R. D. (1970): Carotid endarterectomy for cerebrovascular insufficiency. *Ann. Surg.*, 172:663.
44. Thompson, J. E., Patman, R. D., and Talkington, C. M. (1978): Asymptomatic carotid stenosis: Long-term outcome of patients having endarterectomy compared with unoperated controls. *Ann. Surg.*, 188:308–316.
45. Thompson, J. E., Patman, R. D., and Persson, A. V. (1976): Management of asymptomatic carotid bruits. *Am. Surg.*, 42:77.
46. Treiman, R. L., Foran, R. F., Shore, E. H., and Levin, P. M. (1973): Carotid bruit: Significance in patients undergoing an abdominal aortic operation. *Arch. Surg.*, 106:803.
47. Whisnant, J. P., Matsumoto, H., and Elveback, L. R. (1973): Cerebral ischemia attacks in a community. *Mayo Clin. Proc.*, 48:194–198.
48. Wolf, P. A., Kannel, W. B., McNamara, P. M., et al. (1979): Asymptomatic carotid bruits and risk of stroke. *Stroke*, 10:96.
49. Wylie, E. J., and Ehrenfeld, W. K. (1970): *Extracranial occlusive cerebrovascular disease. Diagnosis and management*, pp. 214–225. W. B. Saunders, Philadelphia.

Controversies in Neurology, edited by R. A.
Thompson and J. R. Green. Raven Press,
New York © 1983.

Cerebral Vascular Disease: Antiplatelet and Anticoagulant Treatment

H. J. M. Barnett

University Hospital, University of Western Ontario, London, Ontario, Canada N6A 5A5

Compelling importance is attached to any treatment or potential treatment for stroke or stroke prevention. This chapter briefly reviews attempts to accredit antithrombotic therapy in the prevention of stroke.

There is a large literature on the subject but a paucity of major and sizable randomized studies using concomitant controls in which both the treatment and the control groups have been accumulated simultaneously and fulfilled the study criteria. A sufficient number of patients are required to give significance to the results of any treatment in a chronic illness with infrequent end-points; usually this requires collaborative multicenter studies, with the alternative of an extension of clinical trials into decades rather than years. Randomization is the only convincing method to avoid selection bias. The balance in each group of the important variables is difficult to achieve but made possible by the randomization process. Historical controls, comparisons with known natural history, and comparison with expected trends in populations are much less convincing. Serious doubt surrounds the reasons why the patients were selected to receive or not to receive the therapy; the improvement in the baseline of effective standard care mitigates against comparison with the past. Exact comparability is always such a great uncertainty when other than randomized control and treatment groups are used that it casts a long shadow over any claimed results. In evaluating antithrombotic therapy, the randomized study must be regarded as the gold-standard.

No large-scale trials in primary stroke prevention have been concluded and published during the past 18 months, but considerable new data has accumulated respecting the mode of action of antithrombotic agents, most particularly the platelet antiaggregants. The attempts to evaluate the antithrombotic agents in stroke and its prevention will be scrutinized critically. It is pertinent, as well, to this discussion to consider the recent publications of two major multicenter myocardial infarction antithrombotic drug trials and one mitral stenosis study. Equivocal results of the coronary studies demand that the differences and similarities between myocardial infarction and cerebral infarction be examined. The question is raised whether or not antithrombotic therapy is more rational for threatened stroke and stroke than it might be for myocardial infarction.

117

RATIONALE FOR ANTITHROMBOTIC THERAPY IN THE OVERALL PROBLEM OF STROKE

Current data suggests that 85% of vascular stroke is of thromboembolic origin with approximately 15% related to hemorrhage (1). These figures are more accurate than previous figures because of the increased accuracy with which new imaging devices can delineate cardiac and brain abnormalities.

The variety of mechanisms responsible for threatened stroke must be kept in the foreground when any new or conventional therapeutic strategies are being planned. Three large subgroups of threatened stroke emerge: 1) those associated with platelet thrombogenesis; 2) those associated with coagulation abnormalities; and 3) those in which alternative mechanisms are of paramount importance.

THREATENED STROKE SIGNIFICANTLY RELATED TO PLATELET THROMBOGENESIS

An arbitrary breakdown of threatened stroke mechanisms involving platelet-fibrin activity is set out in Table 1.

Embolization of the artery-to-artery variety, associated with atherosclerosis in the major arteries, remains the most important mechanism in transient ischemic attack (TIA) and minor stroke. Platelet-fibrin emboli visualized in the retina usually come from the large arteries supplying the brain, but might also result from any of the cardiac mechanisms noted in Table 1, or occur in the uncommon circumstances of thrombocytosis. The visualization of atheromatous debris or isolated cholesterol crystals in the retina or at postmortem in the cerebral arteries confirms an arterial origin for any associated symptoms since the heart is not the site of origin of "bright plaques". Their arterial origin could include the arch of the aorta, but save for the most gross lesions, by present methods this huge organ is beyond the limits of accurate clinical imaging.

TABLE 1. *Varieties of TIA related to platelet-induced thrombosis*

1) Emboli from arteries:	Atheroma Fibromuscular dysplasia

2) Emboli from the heart:	Those identifiable by traditional methods:
	  a) SBE
	  b) Mitral stenosis
	  c) Atrial fibrillation
	  d) MI with mural thrombus
	  e) Prosthetic heart valve

	Those identifiable using newer techniques:
	  a) NBTE
	  b) PMV
	  c) Mitral annulus calcification
	  d) Akinetic segments

3) Thrombocytosis	

Thrombogenesis probably accounts for most of the ischemic events which occur in the patient whose artery is occluded but where symptoms are still occurring beyond the occlusion. Thromboembolism may come from the collateral circulation in the ipsilateral common or external artery upon which the hemisphere is now dependent (2), from within the stump of the internal carotid artery in the neck (3), or occasionally from the intracranial "tail" of the thrombus that has extended upwards into the intracranial portion of the vertebral or the carotid arteries (4).

Careful history taken from patients afflicted with ischemic events indicates that a number of them have experienced these events in rather discrete "flurries." The pathological counterpart which corroborates this intermittency of activity of thrombosis has come from studies of thromboendarterectomy surgical specimens (5,6). In two-thirds of the cases where cerebral ischemic events have occurred within a month of surgery, it has been possible to find thrombi attached to the specimen. On the other hand, if more than a month has elapsed since the last ischemic event, only one specimen in five will be found to have associated thrombi. The timing of the examination will determine the frequency with which one can corroborate thrombogenesis as the factor most important in the production of ischemic symptoms.

The process of thrombosis is not of primary importance in other varieties of stroke and threatened stroke (7). Myocardial infarction may occur from vasospasm more commonly than from thrombosis (8). Vasospasm has no proven significance in stroke in the absence of subarachnoid bleeding in rare "hemiplegic migraine", and possibly in the circumstance of a hypertensive crisis.

REPORTED STUDIES OF PLATELET ANTIAGGREGANT DRUGS

Table 2 outlines the reported results obtained from the use of platelet antiaggregants in a series of patients threatened with stroke.

The first study to be reported was that of Acheson et al. (9) and it was a trial of dipyridamole in patients studied for an average of 24 months. In the first half of the study, the dose used was 400 mg; it later was increased to 800 mg. Negative results were reported. The study was carried out using patients threatened with stroke but also patients who had suffered stroke. There were only 169 cases. The negative results cannot be regarded as a final indication of the lack of benefit that might be obtained in a larger study with this drug.

Of the two large studies utilizing aspirin, the Canadian study (10) entered 585 patients between 1971 and 1977, and the American study (11) entered 179 patients between 1972 and 1975. These studies have been reported in full detail, and the summary in Table 2 supplies the essentials. Male responsiveness was reported in the Canadian study and eventually emerged from the American trial when it was sought retrospectively (12). The German trial involved only 54 cases but the response favoring aspirin in reducing TIA and stroke was positive (13). The Swedish study had no placebo group; they entered 156 cases with TIA or partial nonprogressing stroke into a trial and gave them all 2 months of anticoagulant therapy

TABLE 2. *Controlled trials of platelet antiaggregants in threatened stroke*

Designation of trial	Type of case	Number	Treatment and dose/day	Average period of follow-up (months)	Endpoints	Benefit
Bradford trial (9)	TIA, RIND, Stroke	N = 169 T = 85 C = 84	Dipyridamole 400 mg . . . . 800 mg	14 11	TIA, Stroke, Death	Negative
Canadian trial (10)	TIA, RIND, PNS	N = 585 T = 290 C = 295	ASA 1300 mg, Sulfinpyrazone[a] 800 mg	26	Stroke, Death	Positive—ASA
American trial (11)	TIA, RIND, Stroke	N = 179 T = 88 C = 90	ASA 1300 mg	6	TIA, Stroke, Death	Positive—ASA
German trial (13)	TIA, RIND, PNS	N = 58 T = 29 C = 29	ASA 1500 mg	24	TIA, Stroke	Positive—ASA
AMIS trial (15)	MI	N = 4524 T = 2267 C = 2257	ASA 1000 mg	36	(Stroke)[b]	Positive—ASA
PARIS trial (16)	MI	N = 2026 T = 1620 C = 406	ASA 972 mg, Dipyridamole 225 mg	41	(Stroke)[b]	Positive—ASA
Swedish trial (14)	TIA, RIND	N = 134 AC = 68 ASA + P = 67	ASA 1000 mg + Dipyridamole 150 mg or coumadin	12	TIA, Stroke	"Positive"[d] ASA with dipy-ridamole

[a]Since sulfinpyrazone was no more effective than placebo, these two groups were combined in the analysis.
[b]See text. Patients randomized after myocardial infarction, to study recurrent MI.
[c]No placebo group. AC = anticoagulants; ASA + P = aspirin + persantine.
[d]No single-therapy group.

(14). At the end of this time, 135 patients were randomized to continue on anticoagulants or go on to a trial of aspirin plus persantine. Both groups were said to have benefited by the therapy as judged by historical controls and by the anticipated number of events had they not been treated. The lack of a more convincing comparative group reduces the value of this study.

Neither the AMIS (15) nor the PARIS (16) trials were designed to study stroke-threatened patients. However, in both there was a substantial reduction in the incidence of stroke in the aspirin-treated patients compared to those on placebo. In the PARIS trial both the aspirin and the aspirin/persantine groups had a reduction in stroke incidence compared with the placebo groups, but the differences between the group on aspirin alone and that with persantine did not lend support to the possibility that there is potentiation of aspirin activity by the addition of persantine. Although these coronary trials produced interesting differences favoring aspirin, the benefit did not reach statistical significance.

Methodological arguments about the analysis and interpretation have been forthcoming in respect to these studies. A committee of the F.D.A., Public Health Service of the Department of Health, Education and Welfare, reviewed the evidence from the Canadian and American studies; the following summarizes their recommendations:

> "There is evidence that aspirin is safe and effective for reducing the risk of recurrent transient ischemic attacks or stroke in men who have had transient ischemia of the brain due to fibrin platelet emboli.
>
> "There is no evidence that aspirin is effective in reducing TIAs in women, or is of benefit in the treatment of completed strokes in men or women.
>
> "Patients presenting with signs and symptoms of TIAs should have a complete medical and neurologic evaluation.
>
> "Consideration should be given to other disorders which resemble TIAs.
>
> "It is important to evaluate and treat, if appropriate, other diseases associated with TIAs and stroke, such as hypertension and diabetes" (17).

MAJOR UNSETTLED PROBLEMS IN PLATELET ANTIAGGREGANT THERAPY

The major trials, the smaller trials, and the evidence from the major coronary trials still leave a number of unsettled questions about the use of platelet antiaggregants in stroke prevention. The following appear to be the most important at the present time:

1) *Nonresponders:* Some patients respond indifferently or not at all to aspirin therapy. As previously reported, this included patients who had experienced symptoms that involved both the carotid and the vertebral-basilar territory during the 3 months before they entered the study (7); it included patients who had a large number of lesions demonstrable by angiography in the cerebral arteries, by comparison with those who had only a few. It appears, therefore, that in the more advanced cases there is a low degree of responsiveness to aspirin therapy. Advanced atheroma is subject to such complications as rupture of grumous material from the

plaque into the lumen of the artery, and hemorrhage into the atherosclerotic plaque (18). Both of these phenomena will liberate thromboplastin and be a powerful stimulus to the coagulation cascade. Therapeutic programs which alter platelet function will not be effective under these circumstances.

2) *Female unresponsiveness:* This finding has led to lively discussion. It was corroborated in the American trial, and a trial from Italy has indicated a similar lack of female responsiveness (19). Other studies have been published not involving stroke-threatened patients lending support to this clinical observation (20,21,22). Some interesting experimental work has come from a variety of sources, particularly from the work of Kelton (23), who has been able to demonstrate a reduced thrombogenesis in aspirinated male rabbits compared to aspirinated female rabbits. The female rabbits fared the same as the control of either sex (Table 3). Recent *in vitro* work on sex-related differences, following aspirin therapy, has suggested that these differences may be due to an altered interaction of aspirinated platelets on the vessel wall in the two sexes (24). Another approach has been that of Kakkar who has demonstrated an increase in elderly subjects afflicted with peripheral vascular disease in the protein breakdown products of platelets (25). Both beta thromboglobulin and platelet factor IV were increased with age, and the increase was significantly greater in females than in males. The suggestion has been that the increase was due to an increased female platelet responsiveness to aggregating stimuli. A similar study on a male/female differential in aggregation responsiveness, however, has related this difference to the lower hematocrit and therefore increased plasma volume of females as compared to males, and due to an artefact introduced because of the increased amount of anticoagulant present in the glassware into which the specimens are drawn from the female population, relatively anemic to the male (26).

An intriguing additional possibility explaining the male/female differential has been advanced by Dyken (27). He has reviewed in his own TIA study, as well as in the Canadian and American studies, the prognostic difference between males and females. In every instance, the female prognosis is considerably better than the male prognosis. The suggestion is that the vessel wall prostacyclin is more effective in females than in males and that platelet antiaggregant therapy brings the prognosis in the responsive male to about the level of the nonresponding but prognostically more favored female. This may prove to be part of the explanation of this unexpected phenomenon, but this hypothesis requires more study. The figures for prognosis

TABLE 3. *Annual combined rate of stroke and death (10) for non-aspirin treated patients (N = 289)*

	Stroke or death (%)		
	Both sexes	Males	Females
1 year	13	14	11
2 years	22	24	16
3 years	30	35	16

for the untreated patients in the Canadian study indicate that males are at greater risk than are females (Table 3).

3) It remains to be determined whether patients afflicted with cerebral embolization from cardiac causes are benefited by platelet antiaggregants. There is no data for myocardial infarction as no studies have been carried out; the outpouring of tissue factor might argue against the possible benefit of platelet antiaggregants since the coagulation cascade already would be considerably stimulated. A recent study on the benefit to mitral stenosis patients of sulfinpyrazone will be referred to below, since many were receiving some anticoagulant as well as the platelet inhibitor.

It is tempting but not scientifically accurate to transpose the data from the Canadian and American studies to cardiac patients. On the other hand, these cases were specifically excluded from these trials, and therefore we do not have any facts to back up the presumption that platelet antiaggregants might be of benefit in some patients with cardiac emboli.

4) *Synergism* may exist between some antiaggregants as they behave differently at the molecular level. There are theoretical reasons for believing that persantine may potentiate the benefit of aspirin as a platelet antiaggregant. In patients with clinical manifestations of arterial disease, aspirin and persantine together bring the reduced platelet survival time back to normal, whereas aspirin alone has no effect, and persantine alone has less effect than the combination (28). Furthermore, animal studies have suggested that experimental aggravation of platelet aggregation can be negated by aspirin and persantine together but not by either drug acting alone (29). Until the North American collaborative study on stroke prevention comparing aspirin alone with aspirin and persantine together is completed, no conclusions about clinical benefit from this apparent synergism are possible.

5) The *optimum dose* is under review and the subject of much lively discussion. Theoretical considerations have been advanced to indicate that the optimum dose of aspirin to interfere with platelet function without interfering with the protective effect from the prostacyclin synthesized in the endothelial cells of the vessel wall, would be one aspirin tablet a day, or 3 mg per kg per day. One-half a regular aspirin tablet (160 mg per day) has antithrombotic property (30). This was established in patients afflicted with renal failure who are prone to develop thrombosis in the plastic tubing used to construct the arteriovenous dialysis shunts. Unfortunately this clinical condition is not identical to stroke-threatened TIA patients. Uremic patients have coagulation abnormalities, are anemic, have increased levels of circulating prostacyclin and, in addition, are prone to thrombosis in plastic tubing, not in arteries. The experiment did not attempt to prove that a moderate dose of 4 tablets per day was ineffective in inhibiting thrombosis. In other experimental, but not clinical situations, very high doses (equivalent to ten times the dose used in the stroke trials) have been shown to promote thrombosis (31) and in some observations in human volunteers a reasonably high dose (three times the stroke trial dose) of aspirin (3 to 9 g per day) failed to cause an elevation of the bleeding time (32).

In favor of a moderate dose are three particular arguments. First, all the clinical trials which have shown benefit in stroke prevention have used 1000 to 1300 mg of aspirin per day. No trials have been concluded using a smaller dose. Secondly, a dose of 3.9 g of aspirin per day has been claimed to be effective in a double-blind trial against placebo in protecting patients against venous thromboembolism after knee-replacement surgery (33). Finally, there are two cases in the literature in which a congenital lack of the enzyme cyclooxygenase was determined in the patient (34,35). These patients are thereby comparable to patients who have had thromboxane and prostacyclin production suppressed by aspirin, and both of these metabolites were deficient in the one patient in whom they were measured. Instead of being afflicted with thrombosis, as might be hypothesized, these two patients came under medical observation because of a mild bleeding diathesis.

ANTICOAGULANTS

Three major problems have stood in the way of the clarification of the usefulness or lack of usefulness of anticoagulants in stroke prevention:

1) Modern methodology was absent from the larger trials evaluating them. There simply were not enough patients in any study, randomized or otherwise, to satisfy a modern sample-size calculation. The sample size must take into account the known facts regarding the natural course and the chances of events of an end-point nature each year. The calculation must anticipate the fact that some patients will be unable to tolerate the medication and some, inevitably, will be lost to follow-up. Such problems were not recognized generally when the anticoagulant studies were done. Small numbers may give falsely negative results. By way of illustration the experience of the Canadian Aspirin Study may be cited: There were 24 centers in the trial and the overall results yielded significant benefit favoring aspirin therapy. Seventy-five percent of the cases were entered from 14 centers, and the benefit in each of these 14 centers was consistent with the overall result. There was no benefit from the patients entered from 5 centers although they only contained 10% of the cases. There was a reverse benefit and an apparent worsening compared with the controls by virtue of being on therapy in 15% of the cases from 5 centers. Had the study consisted of a small sample size negative conclusions might have been reached by chance alone.

Any sample-size calculations, as in this aspirin study, must take into account the fact that in TIA patients the best available evidence indicates a 7% chance per year of a stroke and a 4% annual risk of death. Thus 540 cases were judged to be needed if aspirin therapy was to show a significant benefit with a 50% risk reduction over a 5 year period. Comparable calculations were not made for the anticoagulant studies because this need was not so clearly identified at the time that these studies were planned.

In the anticoagulant era the possibility of biasing results without randomization was not completely recognized and few of the studies had the benefit of randomization so that few had acceptable identical controls.

Other methodological needs such as the avoidance of contaminating therapy, the need to have a clear definition of what constituted acceptable cases and what were to be the acceptable end-points were not in clear focus at the time of these early studies. The demand for a complete follow-up was not stressed.

2) The influence of risk factors were not understood nor indeed had all of the risk factors been identified. Consistent plans regarding their treatment were not part of any of the trial plans, nor for that matter were risk factors such as hypertension, which aggravate the risk of anticoagulant treatment, given appropriate attention during some of these studies.

3) The varieties of threatened stroke were not delineated. TIA was regarded as a single entity rather than a group of conditions. Some of the conditions within the genus TIA would not be expected to benefit from antithrombotic therapy and were mixed in because they were not recognized as requiring exclusion from a trial to evaluate this form of treatment.

It is quite certain that no granting agency would flow funds to the investigation processes that were used to evaluate anticoagulant therapy if identical studies were designed and submitted in application in 1981. Despite the problems that beset these trials, however, they are the best available. The balance of this chapter consists of a brief review of what appears to be a reasonable interpretation based upon the published data.

ANTICOAGULANTS IN TIA, PROGRESSING STROKE, AND COMPLETED STROKE

The use of anticoagulants in stroke was extensively reviewed in 1976 under the auspices of the Committee for Stroke Facilities (36). No significant controlled studies have been carried out since that analysis. One or two retrospective analyses and reviews have been published.

In the four randomized TIA studies in the literature no benefit in stroke prevention was recorded. Four nonrandomized studies, by contrast, had claimed benefit. The fifth nonrandomized study published since the 1976 review concerned 47 patients with carotid TIAs and 17 with vertebral-basilar TIAs who were given anticoagulants and compared with 75 carotid patients and 47 vertebral-basilar TIA patients not given anticoagulants (37). There was no indication in the paper of the selection process that was used to place the patients who received the anticoagulants in this treatment cadre nor any indication why those that received no anticoagulants were so treated. The variety of TIA was not discussed. No overall reduction in death occurred but a reduced stroke incidence and overall benefit was claimed for the vertebral-basilar cases. The numbers of course are too small to be meaningful. There were 9 hemorrhages into the brain in the patients receiving anticoagulants.

The conclusions regarding TIA and anticoagulants are based on weak data. On an empirical basis it is reasonable to recommend that when platelet antiaggregants fail, TIA patients be given a trial on anticoagulants for a period of three months. It might appear that this should be recommended particularly if there are many episodes, but the evidence is weak indicating that many as opposed to few TIAs are an extra cause for concern.

Neither anticoagulants nor platelet antiaggregants can be claimed with certainty to have superseded that other unsubstantiated but common treatment—endarterectomy. They may both have a role prior to and after this procedure in selected cases.

2) In regard to progressing stroke there are available data in two randomized and two nonrandomized studies. The randomized studies were full of methodological weaknesses. The definition of "progressing stroke" is far from precise and uniform. There were few patients and the selection process was vague. The evidence is suggestive but not conclusive. It appeared that in one of the randomized studies stroke progress was less although the death rate was not. On empirical grounds one might conclude—and most neurologists would recommend—that anticoagulants should be used for a brief period in the face of a progressing stroke, and most would start with Heparin.

3) In completed stroke there are seven randomized, controlled studies and two nonrandomized studies: one of the latter claimed benefit but the others did not. There appears to be no reason to use anticoagulants in the face of a completed stroke.

ANTICOAGULANTS IN THROMBOEMBOLISM OF CARDIAC ORIGIN

The use of anticoagulants in thromboembolism of cardiac origin was the subject of an excellent and extensive review in September 1980 (38), from which the following important generalities emerged.

(a) It is very obvious that cardiac causes of stroke are for the most part of thromboembolic nature, and there is little doubt that thrombogenesis plays a major role. Thus antithrombotic therapy is a rational consideration.

(b) Recurrent cardiac emboli are very common. Thirty to 40% of patients will have a recurrence within a month, and two-thirds of the patients will have a recurrence within a year after the initial event.

(c) Approximately one stroke in five will now be recognized as of embolic origin.

Emboli in Association with Myocardial Infarction

Within 6 weeks of a myocardial infarction the risk of cerebral embolization is at least 5% as judged by clinical studies. Careful postmortem studies indicate that the patients dying because of myocardial infarction have an incidence of emboli between 45% and 60%, and that half of these at least are to the brain.

Sixty percent of the emboli from myocardial infarction occur within the first 3 weeks. Figures have been given as follows: the first week 11%; the second week 33%; the third week 16%; the fourth week 24%. Thereafter, 6% are expected in the second month and 8% in the third month. These figures are useful guidelines in planning the duration of anticoagulant therapy (39).

In one series of 783 patients with myocardial infarction the incidence of stroke was 1.7%. Where the infarct was large, as is the case in one-third of the patients, the stroke incidence rose to 4.7% (40).

Mural thrombus has been identified in 45% of carefully studied cases dying of myocardial infarction. This tendency to mural thrombosis is found when there is a large infarct, a septal infarct, and an infarction associated with congestive heart failure (41).

In postmortem studies thrombus is contained in 75% of left ventricular aneurysms (42).

The information about anticoagulant usage in patients with myocardial infarction comes from three large studies. A controlled study reported by Wright included 1000 cases (43), and the American Veterans Administration (44) and the British Medical Research Council (45) also sponsored large studies. There was a significant reduction in stroke and an indication that 25% fewer patients on anticoagulants have thromboembolic events. There is negligible information available however about the important question of whether anticoagulant therapy benefits patients who have already experienced the first evidence of embolization. No series, and certainly no controlled study, has been published concerning this aspect of the problem.

With the data available the recommendation would be that anticoagulants should be administered to patients who have had a recent myocardial infarction, provided it was a large infarction, or if it involved the septum, or if there was associated congestive heart failure, or if emboli have already occurred, or if an intracardiac thrombus or an aneurysm is known to be present. The time to administer the anticoagulant is controversial, but in the absence of bloody cerebrospinal fluid, or CT detection of a hematoma or bloody infarction, and of course in the absence of subacute bacterial endocarditis, it is recommended that anticoagulants be administered without delay.

Rheumatic Heart Disease and Cerebral Embolization

The factors to be considered here may be summarized as follows:

(a) The incidence of rheumatic heart disease continues to decline. In Canada, death from rheumatic heart disease has declined 75% in the last 25 years (46).

(b) In the presence of mitral stenosis over a 5 year period, 20% of the patients will have clinical evidence of embolization of which three out of five will involve the brain. Postmortem studies will show 50% with evidence of embolization, and of these, 40% to 50% will involve the brain (38).

(c) Recurrent emboli are common. In various series they have recurred over a varying time period in 30% to 75% of patients. The timing of the recurring emboli in rheumatic heart disease is of importance in management. Thirty percent occur 2 weeks after the initial event, 40% within the first month, and 50% to 65% during the first year (38).

(d) It is remarkable to note that there has been only one randomized study on the subject of anticoagulant therapy in rheumatic heart disease and it yielded negative results (36). This could be meaningless however because there were only 12 patients in the treatment group and 16 in the control group. Many retrospective studies have been done and all the studies had serious design flaws. The suggestion emerges from these imperfectly controlled trials that the patients probably benefit from anticoagulant therapy compared to what might be expected without this therapy. On this basis one is forced to make an empirical decision and to recommend anticoagulant therapy for the patient with rheumatic heart disease who has had an embolic event. The recommended duration of therapy is not known but the usual duration would be indefinite or until a surgical procedure made emboli unlikely to recur. This in turn would be dependent on the development of nonthrombogenic valve replacements.

(e) The question of a combination of platelet antiaggregants and anticoagulants in mitral stenosis has been considered. A recent report on this subject suggests extra benefit from the addition of sulfinpyrazone to anticoagulant therapy (47). A variable number of the patients were given a variable period on anticoagulant therapy. The important improvement appeared to come in the subgroup of patients who had decreased platelet survival time. In this subgroup given sulfinpyrazone, only 2 out of 51 patients had further emboli compared with 16 out of 48 patients who received placebo rather than sulfinpyrazone. This same study should be repeated now using other platelet antiaggregants, and using a uniform protocol in respect to anticoagulants.

(f) Anticoagulants with platelet antiaggregants in patients with prosthetic heart valves have been subjected to several studies. Even the most modern prosthetic heart valves initiate thrombogenesis. The combination of dipyridamole and anticoagulants has been shown to be superior to anticoagulants alone in reducing the incidence of fatal and nonfatal thromboembolism in these patients (48). Aspirin with anticoagulants was studied in one careful double-blind and randomized trial in aortic valve replacement (49). One gram per day of aspirin was compared with placebo and over a 2 year period there was a ninefold reduction in the number of emboli with aspirin and coumadin compared with the control group. The fear of bleeding from the gastrointestinal tract was not realized in this study and 148 patients were treated over a 2 year period. Intracranial hemorrhage was encountered three times in the control and twice in the treated group. No trial has been reported in which platelet antiaggregants alone have been compared with placebo in patients with prosthetic heart valves.

Cardiac Arrhythmias without Myocardial Infarction or Rheumatic Heart Disease

The Framingham Study indicated that the risk of stroke with atrial fibrillation and rheumatic heart disease was 17 times that expected, and even when atrial fibrillation was present without rheumatic heart disease or recent myocardial infarction there was a significant increase in stroke risk, 5.6 times that encountered in the rest of the Framingham population (50).

As well as atrial fibrillation the sick sinus syndrome (sino-atrial node disorder) is now recognized as being seriously embologenic. In one series of 100 cases reported, 16 had emboli, and of these, 15 developed in patients with a combined bradyarrhythmia and tachyarrhythmia syndrome (51). In a parallel observation of 41 patients with bradyarrhythmia plus atrial fibrillation or atrial flutter, the same authors detected an incidence of emboli of 7.3%. The suggestion was made that the impaired atrial function was the key factor in predisposing to an intracardiac thrombosis, and that subsequent tachycardia resulted in an increased risk of stroke.

Patients with atrial fibrillation and with the sick sinus syndrome who have evidence of embolization should receive anticoagulation until the rhythm disorder can be corrected.

CONCLUDING COMMENT

Antithrombotic therapy in stroke prevention requires a lot more careful work. The clinician must bear in mind that there are varieties of stroke which are not related to thrombosis. There are a number of nonthrombotic aspects involved in preventing stroke even when the primary process is one of thrombosis or embolism. This involves risk factor management, especially antihypertensive therapy, cessation of cigarette smoking and the treatment of increased hematocrit and thrombocytosis. The role of endarterectomy and bypass surgery are no more clear than the role of antithrombotic therapy. Some place for these strategies undoubtedly exists but will be covered elsewhere in this volume.

REFERENCES

1. Mohr, J. P., Caplan, L. R., Melski, J. W., Goldstein, R. J., Duncan, G. W., Kistler, J. P., Pessin, M. S., and Bleich, H. L. (1978): The Harvard Cooperative Stroke Registry: A prospective registry. *Neurology*, 28:754–762.
2. Barnett, H. J. M. (1978): Delayed cerebral ischemic episodes distal to occlusion of major cerebral arteries. *Neurology*, 28:769–774.
3. Barnett, H. J. M., Peerless, S. J., and Kaufmann, J. C. E. (1978): "Stump" of internal carotid artery a source for further cerebral embolic ischemia. *Stroke*, 9:448–456.
4. Barnett, H. J. M., and Peerless, S. J. (1981): Collaborative EC/IC Bypass Study—the rationale and a progress report. In: *Cerebrovascular Diseases: Proceedings of the 12th Princeton Conference*, edited by J. Moossy and O. M. Reinmuth, pp. 271–288. Raven Press, New York.
5. Gunning, A. J., Pickering, G. W., Robb-Smith, A. H. T., and Ross Russell, R. (1964): Mural thrombosis of internal carotid artery and subsequent embolism. *Quart. J. Med. New Ser.*, 33:155–195.
6. Harrison, M. J. G., and Marshall, J. (1977): The finding of thrombus at carotid endarterectomy and its relationship to the timing of surgery. *Br. J. Surgery*, 64:511–512.
7. Barnett, H. J. M. (1979): The pathophysiology of transient cerebral ischemic attacks: Therapy with platelet antiaggregants. In: *Medical Clinics of North America*, Vol. 63, edited by W. K. Hass, pp. 649–679. W. B. Saunders, Philadelphia.
8. Maseri, A., L'Abbate, A., Baroldi, G., Chierchia, S., Marzilli, M., Ballestra, A. M., Severi, S., Parodi, O., Biagini, A., Distante, A., and Pesola, A. (1978): Coronary vasospasm as a possible cause of myocardial infarction. *New Engl. J. Med.*, 299:1271–1277.
9. Acheson, J., Danta, G., and Hutchinson, E. C. (1969): Controlled trial of dipyridamole in cerebral vascular disease. *Br. Med. J.*, 1:614–615.

10. The Canadian Cooperative Study Group (1978): A randomized trial of aspirin and sulfinpyrazone in threatened stroke. *New Engl. J. Med.*, 299:53–59.
11. Fields, W. S., Lemak, N. A., Frankowski, R. F., and Hardy, R. J. (1977): Controlled trial of aspirin in cerebral ischemia: *Stroke*, 8:301–316.
12. Gent, M. (1979): Recent intervention studies of platelet suppressant drugs in cerebral ischemia: Methodological aspects. In: *Drug Treatment and Prevention in Cerebrovascular Disorders*, edited by G. Tognoni and S. Garattini, pp. 437–448. Elsevier/North Holland Biomedical Press, New York.
13. Reuther, R., and Dorndorf, W. (1978): Aspirin in patients with cerebral ischemia and normal angiograms or nonsurgical lesions. The results of a double-blind study. In: *Acetylsalicylic Acid in Cerebral Ischemia and Coronary Heart Diseases*, edited by K. Breddin, W. Dorndorf, D. Loew, and R. Marx. pp. 97-106. F. K. Schattauer Verlag, Stuttgart.
14. Olsson, J. E., Brechter, C., Bäcklund, H., Krook, H., Müller, R., Nitelius, E., Olsson, O., and Tornberg, A. (1980): Anticoagulant vs. antiplatelet therapy as prophylactic against cerebral infarction in transient ischemic attacks. *Stroke*, 11:4–9.
15. Aspirin Myocardial Infarction Study Research Group (1980): A randomized controlled trial of aspirin in persons recovered from myocardial infarction. *J. Am. Med. Assoc.*, 243:661–669.
16. The Persantine-Aspirin Reinfarction Study Research Group (1980): Persantine and aspirin in coronary heart disease. *Circulation*, 62:449–461.
17. Excerpt from F.D.A. Drug Bulletin 10:2, February, 1980. Dept. of HEW, Public Health Service, Rockville, Md.
18. Barnett, H. J. M. (1976): Pathogenesis of transient ischemic attacks. In: *Cerebrovascular Diseases*, edited by P. Scheinberg, pp. 1–21. Raven Press, New York.
19. Candelise, L., Landi, G., Perrone, P., Barcchi, M., and Brambilla, G. (1982): A randomized trial of aspirin and sulfinpyrazone in patients with TIA. *Stroke*, 13:175–179.
20. Harris, W. H., Salzman, E. W., Athanasoulis, C. A., Waltman, A. C., and DeSanctis, R. W. (1977): Aspirin prophylaxis of venous thromboembolism after total hip replacement. *New Engl. J. Med.*, 297:1246–1249.
21. Kaegi, A., Pineo, G. F., Shimizu, A., Trivedi, H., Hirsh, J., and Gent, M. (1974): Arteriovenous-shunt thrombosis. Prevention by sulfinpyrazone. *New Engl. J. Med.*, 290:304–306.
22. Linos, A., Worthington, J. W., O'Fallon, W., Fuster, V., Whisnant, J. P., and Kurland, L. T. (1978): Effect of aspirin on prevention of coronary and cerebrovascular disease in patients with rheumatoid arthritis. A long-term follow-up study. *Mayo Clinic Proc.*, 53:581–586.
23. Kelton, J. G., Hirsh, J., Carter, C. J., and Buchanan, M. R. (1976): Sex differences in the antithrombotic effects of aspirin. *Blood*, 52:1073–1076.
24. Kelton, J. G., Carter, C. J., Santos, A., and Hirsh, J. (1980): Sex related differences in platelet function in vivo following aspirin administration. *Circulation*, 62:III:342 (abstr.).
25. Cella, G., Zahavi, J., de Haas, H. A., and Kakkar, V. V. (1979): Beta-thromboglobulin platelet production time and platelet function in vascular disease. *Br. J. Hematol.*, 43:127–136.
26. Kelton, J. G., Powers, P., Julian, J., Boland, V., Carter, C. J., Gent, M., and Hirsh, J. (1980): Sex-related differences in platelet aggregation: Influence of the hematocrit. *Blood*, 56:38–41.
27. Dyken, M. L. (1980): Antiplatelet aggregating agents in transient ischemic attacks and the relationship of risk factors: Total experience of six medical centers. In: *Prophylaxe venöser, peripherer, kardialer und zerebraler Gefäbkrankheiten mit Acetylsalicylsäure*, edited by K. Breddin, D. Loew, K. Überla, W. Dorndorf, and R. Marx. pp. 141–148. F. K. Schattauer Verlag, Stuttgart.
28. Harker, L. A., and Slichter, S. J. (1974): Arterial and venous thromboembolism: Kinetic characterization and evaluation of therapy. *Thrombosis et Diathesis Haemorrhagica (Stuttg.)*, 31:188–203.
29. Honour, A. J., Hockaday, T. D. R., and Mann, J. I. (1977): The synergistic effect of aspirin and dipyridamole upon platelet thrombi in living blood vessels. *Br. J. Experimental Pathol.*, 58:268–272.
30. Harter, H. R., Burch, J. W., Majerus, P. W., Stanford, N., Delmez, J. A., Anderson, C. B., and Weerts, C. A. (1979): Prevention of thrombosis in patients on hemodialysis by low dose aspirin. *New Engl. J. Med.*, 301:577–579.
31. Kelton, J. G., Carter, C., Buchanan, M. R., and Hirsh, J. (1978): Thrombogenic effect of high dose aspirin in injury induced experimental venous thrombosis. *Clinical Res.*, 26:350A.
32. O'Grady, J., and Moncada, S. (1978): Aspirin: a paradoxical effect on bleeding time. *Lancet*, ii:780.

33. McKenna, R., Galante, J., Bachmann, F., Wallace, D. L., Kaushal, S. P., and Meredith, P. (1980): Prevention of venous thromboembolism after total knee replacement by high dose aspirin or intermittent calf and thigh compression. *Br. Med. J.*, 280:514–517.
34. Malmsten, C., Hamberg, M., Svensson, J., and Samuelsson, B. (1975): Physiological role of an endoperoxide in human platelets: Hemostatic defect due to platelet cyclooxygenase deficiency. *Proc. Natl. Acad. Sci. U.S.A.*, 72:1446–1450.
35. Pareti, F. I., Mannucci, P. M., D'Angelo, A., Smith, J. B., Sautebin, L., and Galli, G. (1980): Congenital deficiency of thromboxane and prostacyclin. *Lancet*, i:898–900.
36. Genton, E., Barnett, H. J. M., Fields, W. S., Gent, M., and Hoak, J. C. (1977): Cerebral ischemia: the role of thrombosis and of antithrombotic therapy. Study Group on Antithrombotic Therapy. *Stroke*, 8:150–175.
37. Whisnant, J. P., Cartlidge, N. E. F., and Elveback, L. R. (1978): Carotid and vertebral-basilar transient ischemic attacks: Effect of anticoagulants, hypertension and cardiac disorders on survival and stroke occurrence—a population study. *Ann. Neurol.*, 3:107–115.
38. Easton, J. D., and Sherman, D. G. (1980): Management of cerebral embolism of cardiac origin. *Stroke*, 11:433–442.
39. Bean, W. B. (1938/1939): Infarction of the heart. III. Clinical course and morphological findings. *Ann. Int. Med.*, 12:71–94.
40. Thompson, P. L., and Robinson, J. S. (1978): Stroke after acute myocardial infarction: relation to infarct size. *Br. Med. J.*, 2:457–459.
41. Hellerstein, H. K., and Martin, J. W. (1947): Incidence of thrombo-embolic lesions accompanying myocardial infarction. *Am. Heart J.*, 33:443–452.
42. Juergens, J. L., Edwards, J. E., Achor, R. W. P., and Burchell, H. B. (1960): Prognosis of patients surviving first clinically diagnosed myocardial infarction. *Arch. Int. Med.*, 105:444–450.
43. Wright, I. S., Marple, C. D., and Beck, D. F. (1954): *Myocardial Infarction: Its Clinical Manifestations and Treatment with Anticoagulants. A Study of 1031 Cases.* Grune and Stratton, New York.
44. Veterans Administration Hospital Investigators (1973): Anticoagulants in acute myocardial infarction. Results of a cooperative clinical trial. *J. Am. Med. Assoc.*, 225:724–729.
45. Report of the Working Party on Anticoagulant Therapy in Coronary Thrombosis to the Medical Research Council (1969): Assessment of short term anticoagulant administration after cardiac infarction. *Br. Med. J.*, 1:335–342.
46. Statistics Canada (1980): Causes of death 1978. Catalogue #84–203. Queens Printer, Ottawa, Canada.
47. Steele, P., and Rainwater, J. (1980): Favourable effect of sulfinpyrazone on thromboembolism in patients with rheumatic heart disease. *Circulation*, 62:462–465.
48. Sullivan, J. M., Harken, D. E., and Gorlin, R. (1971): Pharmacologic control of thromboembolic complications of cardiac-valve replacement. *New Engl. J. Med.*, 284:1391–1394.
49. Dale, J., Myhre, E., Storstein, O., Stormorken, H., and Efskind, L. (1977): Prevention of arterial thromboembolism with acetylsalicylic acid. A controlled clinical study in patients with aortic ball values. *Am. Heart J.*, 94:101–111.
50. Wolf, P. A., Dawber, T. R., Thomas, H. E., Jr., and Kannel, W. B. (1978): Epidemiologic assessment of chronic atrial fibrillation and risk of stroke: The Framingham Study. *Neurology (Minneap.)*, 28:973–977.
51. Fairfax, A. J., and Lambert, C. D. (1976): Neurological aspects of sinoatrial heart block. *J. Neurol. Neurosurg. Psychiat.*, 39:576–580.

Controversies in Neurology, edited by R. A.
Thompson and J. R. Green. Raven Press,
New York © 1983.

Some Observations on the Current Management of Arteriovenous Malformations

Sean Mullan

University of Chicago Hospitals, Chicago, Illinois 60637

The treatment of cerebral arteriovenous malformations (AVM) can be the most difficult in neurosurgery. Mortality and morbidity have both been high. To incur high risks may be acceptable in patients who have had one or multiple hemorrhages. It is not acceptable in those whose presenting symptoms are epilepsy or headache. Moderate risks might be assumed in some patients with progressive neurological deficit. Considering the high degree of surgical skill that has been brought to this problem in recent decades, it does not seem likely that a further increase in mere manual surgical skill will eliminate the mortality and morbidity. We must instead seek a better understanding of the problems that these malformations present and devise adjunctive and supplementary strategies to deal with them.

DEFECTIVE AUTOREGULATION OF BLOOD SUPPLY

A syndrome which is becoming increasingly recognized is that of defective autoregulation of the blood supply to the normal brain proximal to the arterial clipping. This leads to the "swollen" or "erect" brain with difficulties due to bleeding at surgery, and to bleeding, swelling, pressure, and displacement problems postoperatively. It is a major cause of both mortality and morbidity. Methods used to reduce this problem include temporary partial clamping of the carotid and staged operative removal. Methods other than direct excision, designed to reduce the spontaneous hazard of malformations while minimizing the interventional risks, are (a) percutaneous embolization by discrete particulate material (3), (b) percutaneous embolization by liquids introduced through an extended intravascular catheter, and (c) operative embolization by liquids introduced into vessels during craniotomy. The present paper relates our experience with several of these methods.

We have described three patients who developed a severe, well documented post occlusion hyperemic or "erect" brain syndrome (1). Two died and one recovered. In the first case, that of an 18-year-old girl, the swelling began acutely after completing the occlusion of the arterial blood supply (anterior and middle) of a right parietal malformation. Serial disruptive cortical hemorrhages occurred in the normal proximal cortex necessitating progressive clipping of the middle cerebral artery. They were finally controlled after the middle cerebral artery was reduced to a pulsating stump deep within the Sylvian fissure.

In a subsequent patient, a 63-year-old woman, an attempt was made to occlude the very large middle cerebral arteries of a giant middle cerebral malformation by inserting large plastic spheres into the carotid artery in the neck. The spheres lodged in the proximal middle cerebral artery and in the syphon. The patient was completely relieved of her long-standing headaches. The next day she had a sudden fatal hemorrhage. The emboli had migrated into the malformation within the Sylvian fissure and an acute hemorrhage had occurred into the external capsule of the normal brain proximal to the malformation.

In the third case—again a giant middle cerebral aneurysm, operated under local anesthesia—a distressing cerebral swelling or erection occurred after placing a ligature on the middle cerebral artery proximal to the malformation. Despite release of the ligature within a few minutes, the swelling persisted for an hour. The patient survived intact.

In all three patients the presenting symptom was chronic headache although patients one and three subsequently bled. Also in all three, the malformation was a giant one, mainly fed by a greatly enlarged middle cerebral artery, although in patients one and three it was also fed by the anterior cerebral.

Since that report, reviewed above, we have had two other patients with a giant parieto-occipital malformation supplied by the middle cerebral artery and also by the vertebral. The fourth patient, a 45-year-old woman, had chronic severe headaches, as did the first three. Patient five, a 51-year-old man, had severe presenting intracerebral hemorrhage. Both of these patients could tolerate manual carotid compression: in both, a common carotid Selverstone clamp was applied and set in the subtotal position with no signs or symptoms of neurological impairment. Both could tolerate preoperative test lowering of the systemic blood pressure from 132 systolic and 136 systolic to 80 systolic and 85 systolic, respectively. Excision of the malformation was carried out in both, uneventfully, at normal blood systolic pressure.

In case 4, there was some obvious "swelling" of the cortex, proximal to ligation, but there was no problem with hemostasis and no operative or postoperative complications. Angiography at 10th and 11th days, respectively, showed a diminution in caliber of the middle cerebral vessels. After 3 days, the clamp was slowly opened, one-fourth turn each day, and removed on the 10th day, respectively. It was believed that this temporary subtotal carotid occlusion had prevented the possibility of serious or even fatal cerebral "swelling" and disruptive hemorrhage.

A sixth patient we saw is more difficult to understand but probably fits into the same category. This 21-year-old man presented with epilepsy. His left occipital malformation had a generous blood supply, but was not considered to be giant in size; nor did his symptoms present as headache. He could tolerate left carotid compression, and since we believed he would not experience a hyperemic problem, partial carotid clamping was not used. An attempt was made to remove the malformation without sacrificing function by keeping very close to the sec. This was accomplished without undue difficulty by coagulating the feeding vessels as they broke up, rather than by clipping the feeding vessels at a distance. Hemostasis was complete, and the patient woke up uneventfully, speaking and moving all limbs.

Within 2 hours, he lapsed into a coma, one pupil dilated. A left subdural hematoma and some blood in the arteriovenous cavity were removed. The brain was not swollen. A small bleeder was seen in the posterior cerebral distribution. Hemostasis was completed. There was evidence of intracranial bleeding again 6 hours later. The cavity was filled with clot, and the cavity margins were swollen and hemorrhagic. After hemostasis was completed, the operating team remained in the operating room for 10 hours with the craniotomy open to make sure that no rebleeding occurred: 6 hours after closing, there was further bleeding which was again removed and observed for a further 4 hours. The patient sustained major left hemisphere damage from which he is slowly improving. Fresh frozen plasma was administered every 30 minutes beginning at the onset of the second opening, and continuing until 1 day after the final reopening. Although the platelet count was never below 100,000, fresh platelets were administered during the last 2 openings and for 2 days thereafter. For 1 week, the blood pressure, which tended to rise, was kept below 150 systolic by nitroprusside. Although the hematology service entertained the possibility of von Willebrand's disease, this could not be substantiated by extensive testing of the patient and his family.

In retrospect, it would appear that the problem could have been averted by the use of the subtotal clamp. It was noted that each time on reopening, ooze was best controlled by a temporary lowering of systolic blood pressure to about 70 mm Hg. Another possible technical aid would have been more proximal control of the major feeding vessels, although this would have endangered the cortex we wished to spare. It might also have permitted more proximal hemorrhagic disruption of tissue, and for that reason, it was not employed until the final (fourth) procedure.

Previously we had anticipated proximal swelling and hemorrhagic disruption if the patient had a giant AVM fed by the middle cerebral artery, and especially if he presented with headache. This experience makes us wonder if this protection should also be made available to the moderate AVM patient. Even if an experience such as this occurs only once, it would be worthwhile to have a clamp always available since the clamp itself should be a no-risk procedure. Alternatively, efforts should be made to determine preoperatively which patients are prone to loss of proximal autoregulation. Pertuiset *(personal communication)*, has suggested that the reaction of blood volume to induced hypotension might prove helpful. In this test, the volume of blood in the AVM normally decreases, and that in the brain increases indicating that the latter is capable of expansion and contraction. Those patients in whom the brain vessel volume is already maximally expanded would be expected to sustain disruption once the AVM was clipped. However, it would seem that this test would only identify the most distressed situations, and would not identify patients such as case 6. Intraoperative pressure, recording of the proximal vessels before and after occlusion, might prove helpful in determining whether or not to use a previously implanted carotid clip.

MANAGEMENT OF DIFFICULT AVMs

There is another group of difficult AVMs—those situated on or close to the medial surface of the brain, on or near the motor strip, and supplied by the anterior, middle, and posterior cerebral arteries. Embolization of the vertebral and middle cerebral components will reduce the bulk of the lesion considerably, and it can be done slowly and safely in a multistaged procedure. However, because of the angle of origin of the anterior cerebral artery, it can rarely be embolized. Its sudden occlusion by operation after the middle and posterior cerebral arteries have been embolized might suddenly reduce the total hemispheric blood supply below the critical level with resulting neural deficiency.

It is therefore desirable to occlude the anterior cerebral first. Mere ligature is followed by early collateral revascularization. We have had experience with the occlusion of the anterior cerebral artery by cyanoacrylate inserted by craniotomy in eight such malformations.

It was found that the use of a needle was unsatisfactory in that (a) it could penetrate the opposite wall of the injected pericallosal or callosal marginal artery, or (b) it could be ejected from the artery by the injection pressure once the cyanoacrylate began to harden distally. We have found that the most useful method consists of penetrating the arterial branch by a Number 21 intra-arterial plastic catheter. It is then hooked to a two-way stopcock and two 1.0 ml syringes. One contains 5% glucose. The other contains 1.0 ml of liquid cyanoacrylate. The glucose is used to flush the needle and the artery. Hardening of the cyanoacrylate does not occur in the presence of a nonionic solution such as glucose. However, once it comes in contact with an ionic solution (NaCl or tissue fluid), it hardens in a few seconds. Usually, this is about 7 seconds in tissue fluid, but it may take 30 to 60 seconds to harden within an artery which has just been flushed out by glucose. Although pantopaque can mix with cyanoacrylate, and can both slow the hardening, and show the volume of deposit, we have not used it because of the variation in the hardening time it introduced. In general, we used 1.0 ml per arterial branch (pericallosal and callosomarginal) but sometimes used less as hardening occurred. A rapid injection could push several milliliters through before hardening occurred. The rate of injection was empirical. Although an effort was made to place the injection catheter close to the AVM, this was not always possible because of the access permitted by the venous distribution. If stereoscopic angiography showed a vessel going to what was presumed to be motor cortex, that branch was spared.

There were four patients with a large AVM on the medial surface. None sustained any neurological deficit despite the proximity to the leg-motor area. Angiography after 1 year showed that the occlusion initially reached was sustained.

A fourth patient had a larger malformation which extended out into the central white matter. He developed weakness in his leg 24 hours after surgery. Hemiplegia and aphasia were complete on the fifth day and had cleared by the tenth day.

Three other patients had more laterally situated malformations involving more of the middle cerebral distribution. Two had weakness of the arm, one of the leg;

two had bled previously; and one had a steal. After injection of the pericallosal and callosomarginal arterial branches, two developed predominant weakness of the arm. One developed subtotal hemiplegia and dysphasia. The symptoms cleared in two of the patients in about 3 weeks. In the third a minimal increase in leg weakness over preoperative leg weakness persists. In each case, the onset was delayed, but commenced within 24 hours of surgery.

It would therefore appear that medially situated AVMs are not liable to post-injection neurological deficit, but that those extending deeply into the white matter and those with a previous weakness are liable to weakness. The late onset of the weakness and its total or virtually total resolution suggests that it is not due to vascular occlusion. Whether it represents reactive swelling in the white matter to the thrombus in the AVM, or whether it represents "toxic" leakage from the cyanoacrylate is not known. Its resolution would appear to favor the former. We have not subsequently thrombosed the residual middle cerebral and posterior cerebral feeders in any of these patients, and we do not have immediate or definite plans to do so. Our experience would, however, suggest the staged thrombus by operative injected cyanoacrylate as a possibility.

Intravascular Thrombosis

We have had experience with intravascular thrombosis in two further patients. One sustained a subarachnoid hemorrhage and had some numbness in the right side of his face. He was shown to have a large AVM in the floor of the medulla and to the right of the medulla, which was supplied by a single branch from the right vertebral artery, arising proximal to the right PICA. A triple lumen balloon catheter was inserted into the right vertebral artery so that the balloon lay between the abnormal artery and the PICA. Injection of contrast media through the distal lumen opacified the PICA. Injection through the proximal part gave pain in the right face and opacified the AVM. Injection of saline, and to a lesser extent glucose, also gave pain. Injection of 0.75 ml of cyanoacrylate gave a burning pain in the right face. The AVM and the proximal vertebral artery were obliterated. Subsequently, a left vertebral angiogram showed normal filling of both PICAs. This patient developed a mild Wallenberg syndrome and a severe hiccup. The latter took 3 weeks to subside.

Our final patient in this series with a subarachnoid hemorrhage was shown to have a tentorial-falx AVM which filled a greatly distended vein of Galen. It was filled by the left superficial temporal and middle meningeal arteries, by the left occipital artery, and by both posterior meningeal arteries, and by the tentorial branches of the left meningohypoposeal artery. All of these arteries were directly injected with cyanoacrylate except the tentorial branches of the meningeal artery. The latter was divided and they were obliterated by coagulation.

MANAGEMENT OF INACCESSIBLE AVMs

A third group of patients has interested us, in whom the AVM is situated in the motor strip, or eloquent brain, or in a relatively inaccessible area such as the choroidal fissure, where operative treatment is fraught with a high morbidity. We have attempted to control symptoms in these by silastic embolization, even though total obliteration was not possible. Our methods of percutaneous injection of these emboli, previously described (2), has now been used to treat 40 patients.

This method differs from that of Lussenhop, the pioneer of this type of embolization. His use of relatively large emboli may block arteries proximally and could result in the type of fatal hemorrhage described in the first section of this paper due to swelling or erection of the proximal brain. The smaller emboli which we use penetrate deeper into the malformation in an attempt to obliterate the bed. However, if the reticulum is wide they simply pass through. We have found that if the combined number of arterial feeders exceeds the combined number of draining veins, and if the combined diameter of the arteries exceeds the combined diameters of the veins, then the situation is suitable for embolization, but not vice versa. A number ratio of 5 to 1 and a diameter ratio of at least 2 to 1 appears very favorable. The results of this study will not be known for many years since the natural history is long. Presumably the treatment will have no effect on epilepsy, although it has been quite effective for headache. We have not used it primarily for ischemia. The major problem in determining its indications lies in rebleeding. Three of our patients have rebled during the follow-up. One had a subsequent operative excision, and two, in whom the AVMs presented in the ventricular cavity, rebled and died despite what appeared to be a very satisfactory, nearly complete embolic obliteration. The conclusion at the moment, therefore, is that AVMs which present in the ventricle are not protected by this type of embolization. Information is not yet available regarding the protection afforded AVMs which are strictly cortical in location.

CONCLUSION

On the basis of this experience we feel that some immediate needs in the management of arteriovenous malformations are (a) improvement in predicting the operative and postoperative hyperemic state, (b) a better intraoperative arterial thrombogenic agent than cyanoacrylate, and (c) additional exploration of the role of balloon catheters and liquid thrombogenic agents for use by the percutaneous method.

REFERENCES

1. Mullan, S., Brown, F. D., and Patronas, N. J. (1979): Hyperemic and ischemic problems of surgical treatment of arteriovenous malformations. *J. Neurosurg.*, 51:757–764.
2. Mullan, S., Kawanaga, H., and Patronas, N. (1979): Microvascular embolization of cerebral arterio-venous malformation. *J. Neurosurg.*, 51:621–627.

Controversies in Neurology, edited by R. A.
Thompson and J. R. Green. Raven Press,
New York © 1983.

Guidelines for Management and Surgical Treatment of Intracranial Aneurysms

John M. Tew, Jr.

Mayfield Neurological Institute, Cincinnati, Ohio 45220

The history of the modern treatment of intracranial aneurysms is relatively brief and is known to those surgeons who care for patients with subarachnoid hemorrhage today. Since the publication of the original paper by Sir Charles Symonds (59) in 1924 describing subarachnoid hemorrhage, there has been continuing controversy concerning the merits of medical versus surgical management. The principal method of early surgical treatment was proximal ligation of the carotid artery, although Dott (11) and Dandy (9) had described direct intracranial approaches in 1933 and 1944. The development of angiography, the improvement of anesthetic techniques, and the recognition of the high incidence of recurrent hemorrhage and cerebral ischemia associated with proximal ligation, stimulated the further development of intracranial aneurysm surgery (12).

Paralleling the improved surgical techniques, there occurred increasing awareness of the complex clinical and pathological problems related to subarachnoid hemorrhage from aneurysms. Experience with early surgical treatment was disappointing. Cerebral edema, inadequate exposure and illumination vision, and propensity to uncontrollable rupture, made surgery of the aneurysm a formidable procedure. All too frequently, neurological deterioration of an obscure nature developed several days after apparently successful early clipping of ruptured aneurysms.

SURGICAL VERSUS NONSURGICAL MANAGEMENT

Documentation of the nature of the delayed onset and devastating character of arterial vasospasm is attributable to Crompton (8) who, in 1964, demonstrated the infarction changes which occur at a distance from the aneurysm. Allcock and Drake (3) in 1965 correlated postoperative angiography with the clinical course of deteriorating patients. Their work increased effort along pharmacological and mechanical lines designed to counteract or prevent cerebral vasospasm. Furthermore, Drake's 1965 study motivated a consensus toward delaying the surgical treatment of ruptured aneurysms. Although many patients deteriorated during the waiting period as a consequence of recurrent hemorrhage or other ischemic complications of vasospasm, these consequences were acceptable because the results of delayed surgical treatment were so superior. Since the beginning of surgical treatment of aneurysms, there has been a body of opinions that hold that surgical treatment has no advantage over medical treatment (29,54). This opinion was the principal reason for the randomized study. This national, multicenter study completed in 1969 (46) compared the results of bed rest, hypotensive therapy, and surgical therapy. The conclusion evolved that nonsurgical therapy augmented by bed rest and hypotension was preferable. However, surgeons contended that pooling of data from multiple centers and the varying nature of surgical procedures obscured the good results of selective procedures. This study revealed no single mode of treatment to be superior to others for all aneurysm sites and under all circumstances of patient condition, age, and elapsed time from subarachnoid hemorrhage (SAH). A combination of factors, but especially the patient's condition after hemorrhage, was considered to have a greater influence on survival than the differences among treatments themselves. Although clipping of the aneurysm removes the threat of recurrent hemorrhage with acceptable certainty and restores normal life expectancy and freedom of action, according to the criteria of the study, carotid ligation was a superior treatment. Subsequent studies by Jane (24) indicate that patients with posterior communicating aneurysms treated by carotid ligation are protected from recurrent SAH for only 1 year. Thereafter, rebleeding occurs with the same frequency in treated and untreated individuals.

Conclusions gleaned from the cooperative study indicated that progress in management of the patient with an aneurysm would best be served if improvements and innovations in the techniques of surgical attack could reduce the risks of surgical mortality and morbidity. Prior to 1969, these acceptable surgical results could be achieved in 90% of surgical candidates if the operative procedure was delayed 2 weeks or more from the date of the last SAH, and if the patient was in excellent condition. The study also indicated the desirability of preventing rebleeding until the patient's condition improved to a state when surgical treatment could be applied with relative safety. The need was cited for a regimen to prevent progressive cerebral ischemia due to arterial vasospasm. The major thrust of effort during the last decade has been directed toward solving these three challenges.

MICROSURGERY

The greatest single technical advance in treatment of intracranial aneurysms has been the development of microsurgery. Sir Edward S. R. Hughes said that microsurgery was the most spectacular advance in surgery in modern times. The American College of Surgeons ranked the application of microsurgery in the treatment of cerebrovascular disease among the first order of research advances between 1945 and 1970 (43). This new technique came at an opportune moment for the neurosurgeon. The improved illumination, magnification, and mobility provided by the surgical microscope were enhanced by improved instrumentation, techniques for reducing brain volume, systemic hypotension, and the skill of advancing neuroanesthetic practices. Minute anatomic details can be unraveled by meticulous and precise dissection with delicate, sharp instruments. Hypotension permits the aneurysm to be dissected, manipulated, and clipped with precision that defies imagination. A new surgical science was heralded by the publication of the monograph by Yasargil in 1969 (62). Pupils from all over the world traveled to Zurich to observe a technique that has lowered the mortality figures in aneurysm surgery to negligible levels.

RECURRENT HEMORRHAGE AND ARTERIAL VASOSPASM

These technical innovations did not solve the critical problems related to recurrent hemorrhage and arterial vasospasm, although the question of timing in planning surgical treatment was raised again as a substantive issue. Yasargil discounted vasospasm as a relevant concern but reserved the decision to delay surgical treatment for patients in poor clinical condition (63,26). A decade earlier, Pool (41) had suggested that early surgery might neutralize vasospasm and eliminate rebleeding. More recently, Hunt (21,22) and Sampson (52) have advocated early surgery and report no deaths in Grade I and II patients (Table 1). Saito (47,48) and Suzuki (58) report no mortality and minimal morbidity in Grade I and II patients operated within 2 to 3 days following SAH. However, Drake (12) continues to recommend delay for at least 7 days after SAH and proceeds with surgery only if the patient is neurologically stable and has no vasospasm. Mullen (31) has achieved a zero operative mortality and minimal morbidity in low-risk patients by intensive use of regional and systemic hypotension, antifibrinolysin, and delayed surgery. Sundt (57) advisedly has recommended that there is no ideal time for surgical treatment. These divergent opinions from acknowledged authorities accent the complexity of the timing issue, and probably indicate that there are no simple prognostic factors which permit the clinician to choose the correct date for the clipping of an aneurysm. In an effort to resolve the dilemma, a multicenter collaborative study has been designed to determine whether early operation with removal of fresh clot will have a salutory effect on the disturbing frequency of ischemic disasters and simplify the complex management problems. Recent studies (10,14) indicate that the computerized scan may provide a highly reliable prognostic indicator of the clinical course following SAH from intracranial aneurysm. Absence of blood or minimal localized blood on CT scan within 72 hours of SAH appears to be a reliable indicator that clinically significant vasospasm is a remote risk, whereas diffuse subarachnoid blood and/or parenchymatous hematoma is associated with a serious risk of clinical deterioration even if the initial clinical condition is good (14). Fisher (16) reported

TABLE 1. *Classification of patients with intracranial aneurysms according to surgical risk*

Grade I:	Asymptomatic, or minimal headache and slight nuchal rigidity
Grade II:	Moderate to severe headache, nuchal rigidity, no neurological deficit other than cranial nerve palsy
Grade III:	Drowsiness, confusion, or mild focal deficit
Grade IV:	Stupor, moderate to severe hemiparesis, possible early decerebrate rigidity and vegetative disturbances
Grade V:	Deep coma, decerebrate rigidity, moribund appearance

Adapted from Hunt and Hess.

that severe vasospasm was *almost* never encountered when subarachnoid blood was not detected or only faintly distributed. Severe vasospasm almost invariably occurred (23 of 24 cases) in the presence of large subarachnoid clots layered in fissures and cisterns. Furthermore, there was a precise relationship between the location of blood clots and the site of vasospasm (Figs. 1 and 2).

We submit that the CT scan may provide a critical prognostic indication for early operation if subarachnoid blood is minimal or absent. Our experience also indicates that rebleeding is infrequent in these patients and in most instances they can be easily nursed for 6 to 7 days with minimal difficulty. Conversely, in patients with localized thick subarachnoid clots or parenchymatous hematoma, it may be prudent to operate within the first 48 hours, remove the maximal amount of clot, clip the aneurysm, and direct the subsequent therapy toward prevention of ischemic complications. The role of early surgery in diffuse, layered subarachnoid blood continues to be controversial despite the enthusiasm of our colleagues from Japan (47,48,58).

The indications for early operation include: (a) prevention of rebleeding, (b) prevention of ischemic complications of vasospasm (if removal of focal or diffuse hematoma is effective), (c) application of current therapeutic measures to treat vasospasm without concern for recurrent hemorrhage, (d) removal of life-threatening hematoma, and (e) definitive clipping of aneurysms in the face of rapidly recurring hemorrhage. The most forceful argument for early surgery in the patient with a major SAH (i.e., Grade I and II patients with marked SAH on CT scan) is removal of the aneurysm as a source for rebleeding. Thereafter, the most current and promising panacea, volume expansion and controlled hypertension, can be implemented without fear of fatal rebleeding. This concept is untested since the reported results of early surgery are largely anecdotal and have not been subjected to random study.

A multinational cooperative study, developed at the University of Iowa, has been initiated and will provide an opportunity for critical analysis of timing and control of the factors judged to be crucial in the management of patients with SAH. This study should illuminate the natural history of SAH due to aneurysmal rupture since only patients admitted to the hospital and studied within 3 days of a single SAH will be included. Reports available from the recently completed cooperative aneurysm study, Phase V (J. C. Thorner, 1979, *unpublished data*), the New York University (42), the Mayo Clinic (57), and the University of Chicago (31), provide some interesting and alarming insights into the problems of managing patients with SAH. The 1,018 patients were treated in diverse manner with highly variable results. The survival rate was uniform at nearly 80% but morbidity appeared to be determined by the nature of the hospital practice. In the cooperative study group where patients were admitted to a recording center at an early date, the mortality and morbidity was uniformly greater. Of particular note, the overall survival of 64% and favorable outcome of 43% was recorded in 249 patients admitted to the study less than 72 hours after SAH. These findings appear to be realistic; in fact they are nearly identical with those of a recent retrospective study of 75 patients with acute SAH in our two university hospitals (Tables 2 and 3).

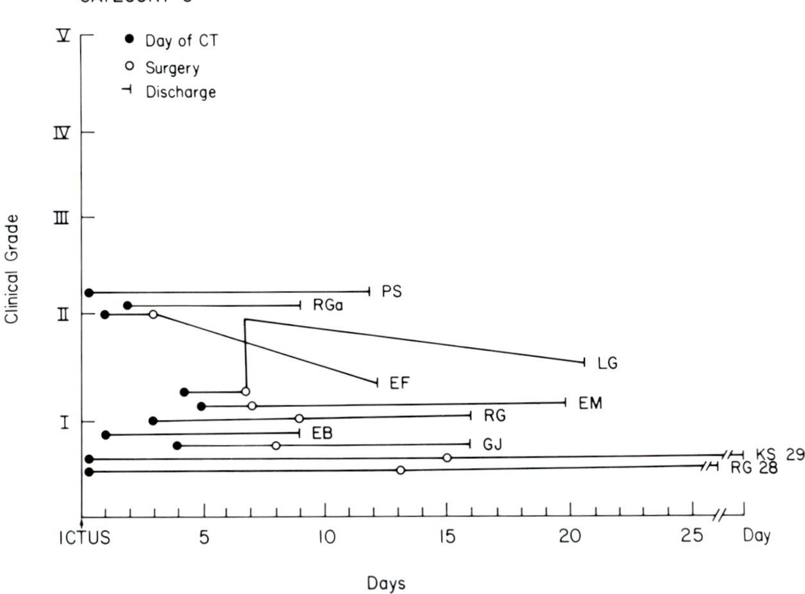

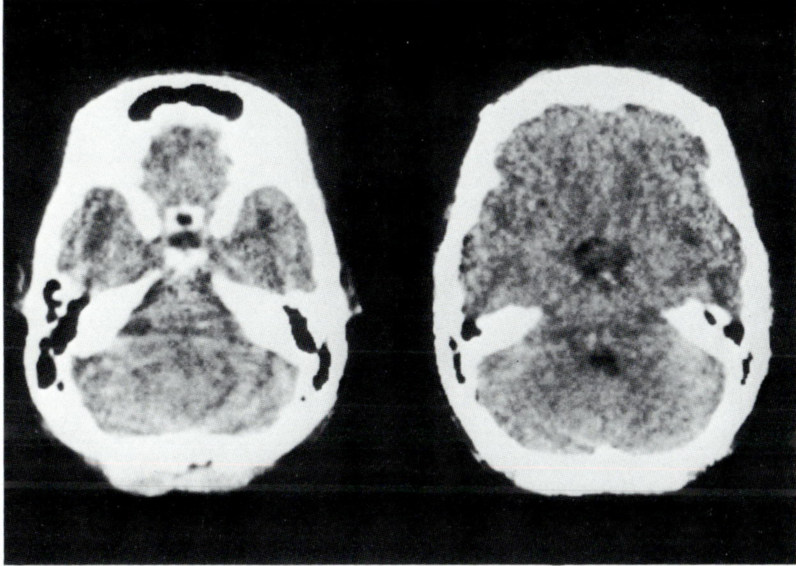

FIG. 1. CT scan—category 0. **Top**: No blood and clinical course which is uniformly benign in 10 patients. **Bottom**: CT scan—category 0. No evidence of blood 24 hours after SAH and third nerve palsy.

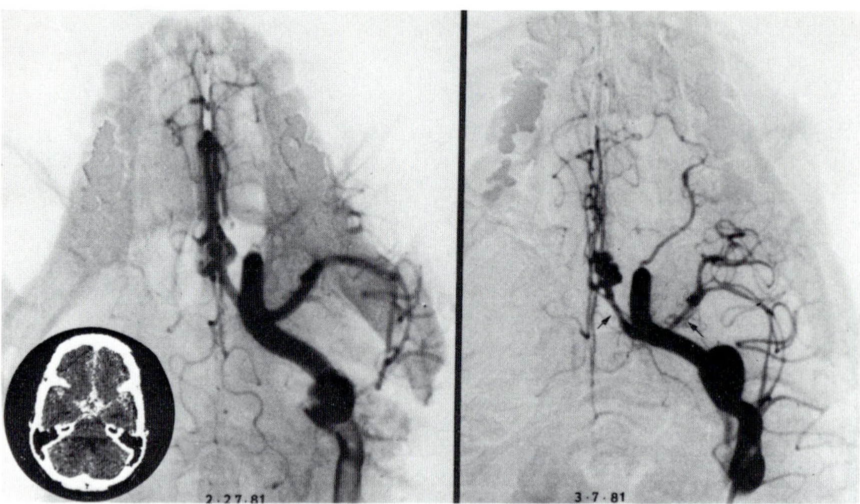

FIG. 2. CAT scan—category 1. Diffuse subarachnoid hemorrhage of marked degree is associated with high incidence of deterioration due to vasospasm. Deterioration of grade is seen even in most good patients. Lack of spasm on 2/27/81 **(left)** and marked spasm 8 days later on 3/7/81 **(right)**. Clinical deterioration was evident as depressed consciousness and hemiparesis.

TABLE 2. *Management of intracranial aneurysms*

	Cooperative study Phase V	N.Y.U.	Mayo Clinic	U. of Chicago
No. of cases	511	100	310	97
Time of admission	0–7	0–>40	<31	?
Neurological status "good" on admission	80%	43%	71%	56%
Percent operated	66%	86%	90%	71%
Neurological status "good" at surgery	89%	58%	68%	100%
Timing of surgery (days)	16+	4–>40	>9	>10
Operative mortality	10%	8%	5%	0%
Rebleeding	10%	12%	14%	6%
Overall survival	71%	85%	86%	85%
Overall favorable outcome	48%	60%	73%	84%

In the important report by Mullen (31) on the management of 97 patients (U. of Chicago, Table 2), the operative mortality was zero (71% of patients were operated upon, all more than 10 days after SAH), rebleeding was held to 6%, the overall survival and favorable outcome was 85%. Mullen attributes the rarity of recurrent hemorrhage to aggressive antifibrinolytic therapy and effective blood pressure control. Few have been as successful or as diligent as Mullen in using the treatment he recommends. Conflicting reports (53) concerning the effectiveness of antifibri-

TABLE 3. *Cooperative study of aneurysms, Phase V*

No. of cases	249	262	511
Time of admission	0–3	4–7	0–7
Neurological status "good" on admission	76%	84%	80%
Rebleeding	13%	7%	10%
Percent operated	65%	66%	66%
Neurological status "good" at surgery	88%	89%	89%
Timing of surgery (days)	16+	16+	16+
Operative mortality	12%	8%	10%
Overall survival	64%	76%	71%
Overall favorable outcome	43%	53%	48%

nolytic therapy and potential side effects (5,40) have deterred uniform acceptance of the regimen advocated by the National Institutes of Health (NIH) cooperative study which was completed in 1975 (32). The report demonstrated a 50% reduction in rebleeding in patients treated with epsilon-aminocaproic acid (EACA). Mullen (31) controls arterial blood pressure by administering intravenous agents (Arfonad or nitroprusside), and regional blood pressure by using partial carotid clamping. The blood pressure is titrated downward until general or regional ischemic symptoms appear. The pressure is then elevated 15 mm or to a figure 30% lower than the initial pressure. This approach has had to be abandoned in a few patients because of neurological deterioration of ischemic nature. Partial carotid occlusion to achieve regional control of pressure, a concept conceived by Mullen (31), has been associated with a high incidence of complications. Although the idea has merit for aneurysms of the internal carotid and middle cerebral arteries, it has not gained wide application.

NATURAL HISTORY OF INTRACRANIAL ANEURYSMS

Despite the advances of microsurgery and therapeutic management, many problems remain unsolved. The natural history of intracranial aneurysms has been clarified by recent studies. Jane (24) concluded that approximately 65% of patients die in the first bout of SAH and many of them have not seen a physician. He concluded that since most patients are not subjected to surgical treatment in less than 14 days, the critical aspects of natural history begin at 2 weeks: (a) Rebleeding progressively decreases in frequency until the incidence becomes static at about 6 weeks, but rebleeding from anterior circulation aneurysms continues after 6 months at a rate of 3 to 4% annually, and the cumulative mortality rate from recurrent hemorrhage is 67%; (b) advanced age, higher clinical grades, and arterial hypertension are associated with significantly greater risk for hemorrhage; and (c) anatomic configuration, size, location, and size change are factors influencing rebleeding. Jane's findings support the rationale for operating on all aneurysms that have ruptured regardless of the time elapsed since SAH, if other clinical factors are in agreement.

Drake (12) concluded that surgeons probably have a beneficial impact on only 1 of 6 patients with aneurysmal hemorrhage. His conclusion was based on statistics from epidemiological studies from Japan (33), Canada (12), and the United States (40) which indicate that only 1 to 3 patients with aneurysms per 100,000 population are operated annually (the favorable outcome is 50 to 70%) while the incidence of SAH remains relatively constant at 11 to 13 per 100,000 per year.

Alarming confirmatory data can be found in the study of Phillips et al. (40) at the Mayo Clinic, who documented the "Unchanging Pattern of Subarachnoid Hemorrhage in a Community." The community of Rochester, Minnesota, allowed the opportunity to examine all cases of SAH for a 30-year period. The incidence was constant at 11 per 100,000 per year. The onset increased with age (the median was 58 years) documenting the acquired nature of SAH due to aneurysmal lesions.

The probability of surviving for 30 days after the first SAH was only 42% (Fig. 3), a finding which was similar to Pakarinen's study from Finland (37). A trend toward better survival has occurred since 1970, but the difference is not statistically significant despite the availability of advanced diagnostic, therapeutic, and surgical techniques (only 8% of patients failed to attain medical attention). The probability of survival was related closely to clinical grade (Fig. 4), the time after the SAH (Fig. 5), and the occurrence of rebleeding. The probability of rebleeding was maximal in 10 days (20%), peaked by 20 days, and became relatively constant after 30 days. Rebleeding occurred at a rate of 1.5% per year for the first 10 years. This important study documents the disastrous natural history of SAH due to ruptured intracranial aneurysm, a course which is largely unaltered by the best medical and surgical care because of the pitfalls in diagnosis (1) and the nature of the disease (27,61,64).

The documentation of the devastating nature of SAH comes at a time when we have the technology to demonstrate the presence of unruptured aneurysms in the population at risk. McCormick (28) found aneurysms in 7.8% of consecutive nec-

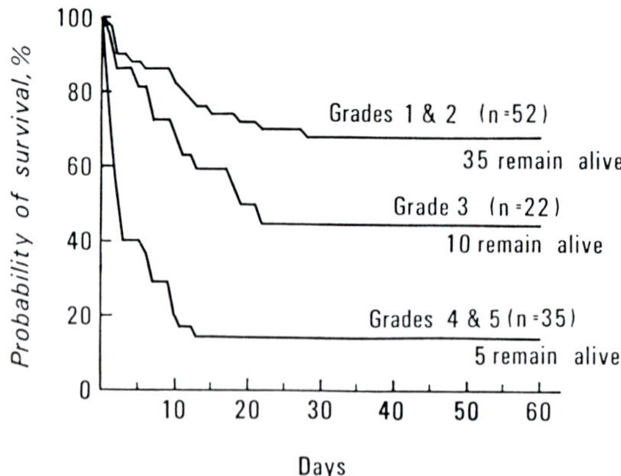

FIG. 3. Probability of survival related to time after hemorrhage and the year of hemorrhage. (From Phillips et al., ref. 40, with permission.)

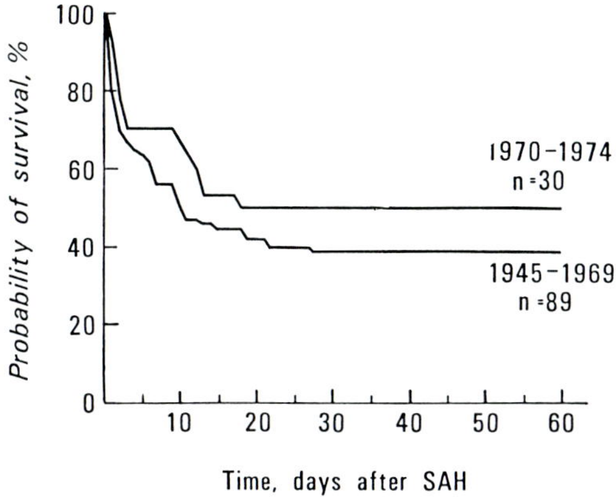

FIG. 4. Probability of survival related to clinical grade and time after hemorrhage. (From Phillips et al., ref. 40, with permission.)

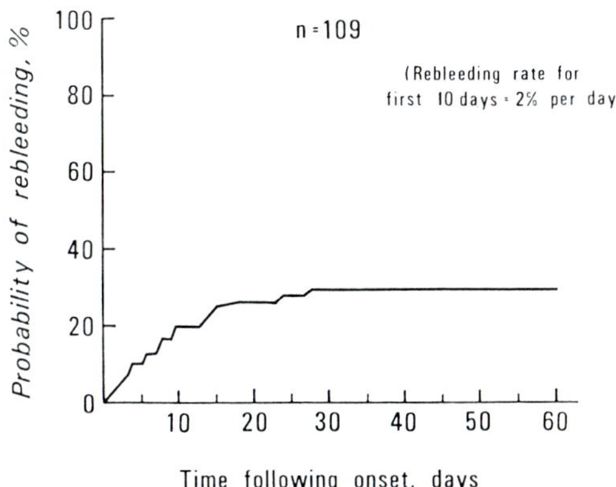

FIG. 5. Probability of rebleeding related to time following onset of hemorrhage. (From Phillips et al., ref. 40, with permission.)

ropsies. The incidence increased progressively through the sixth decade. He estimates that 20% of aneurysms rupture during life and that size has a profound influence on the risk of rupture. Allcock (2) documented angiographically that aneurysms enlarge during life, and Jane (24) proved the greater incidence of bleeding with enlargement. Several recent developments allow for the screening of patients who are suspected to have had SAH or who have an asymptomatic aneurysm. Iron positive cells may appear in the cerebrospinal fluid (CSF) up to 17 weeks after SAH, establishing the prior occurrence of SAH when the CSF is no longer bloody or xanthochromic (23). Among the rare studies concerning the determination of the population at risk for rupture of an aneurysm, Okawara's analysis (35) of warning signs is outstanding. He found three distinct groups of signs: (a) *Headache*, presumed to be vascular in origin, was attributed to expansion of the aneurysm or adjacent artery, occurred in 65% of patients, and was present for an average of 110 days prior to rupture. Fifty percent of patients had localized headache. (b) *Minor or warning bleeding* occurred in 50% of patients on an average of 10 days prior to major hemorrhage. (c) *Ischemic lesion due to arterial spasm or cerebral emboli* occurred in 20% of patients on an average of 21 days prior to major hemorrhage (Table 4).

We have had meager experience with the relationship between ischemia and delayed hemorrhage. In fact, we have not observed a single patient in whom distal embolization from an aneurysm has been followed by rupture. In other reports (4,15,20,49,56) there is no documented association, a finding which may be attributable to the stasis and thrombus which are frequently observed in aneurysms associated with distal embolization (44). Gillingham (17,18) first called our attention to the "warning leak" which in his opinion occurred in 70% or more instances of ruptured aneurysm—a warning which frequently goes unrecognized by patient and physician until the opportunity to alter the course is lost to a calamitous recurrent hemorrhage. Okawara's report confirms the opinion of Gillingham and King (25) of the importance of the warning leak establishing the significance of headache of long duration prior to SAH. King reported that headache was a warning symptom in 60% of patients; it was intense and unusual for 6 months in nearly half of the patients studied. Therefore, headache of an unusual nature, localized or generalized, should be considered a forewarning of SAH.

There are several other conditions which are associated with intracranial aneurysm. (a) Polycystic renal disease: In nearly 20% of cases, this disorder is associated with single or multiple aneurysms, and SAH is a common cause of death in patients with this malady (6).

(b) Coarctation of the aorta: Twelve percent of patients with coarctation of the aorta die of intracranial hemorrhage which in most reported cases has been due to ruptured aneurysm (60).

(c) Fibromuscular dysplasia (FMD): Cerebral aneurysms have been found in many patients with fibromuscular dysplasia of the extracranial arteries. In our experience, the incidence of aneurysm is 20%. There is some controversy concerning the genetic etiology; Palubinskas (38) reported the coexistence of FMD of carotid arteries and cerebral aneurysm in 50% of patients.

(d) Ehlers-Danlos syndrome (pseudoxanthoma elasticum), Marfan's syndrome, aortic stenosis and atresia, connective tissue disorders, and congenital defects are all associated with a heightened risk of cerebral aneurysm (45).

TABLE 4. *Warning signs of aneurysmal rupture*

1. Headache (65%)—110 days
2. Ischemic lesion (20%)—21 days
3. Warning hemorrhage (60%)—10 days

From Okawara, ref. 35, with permission.

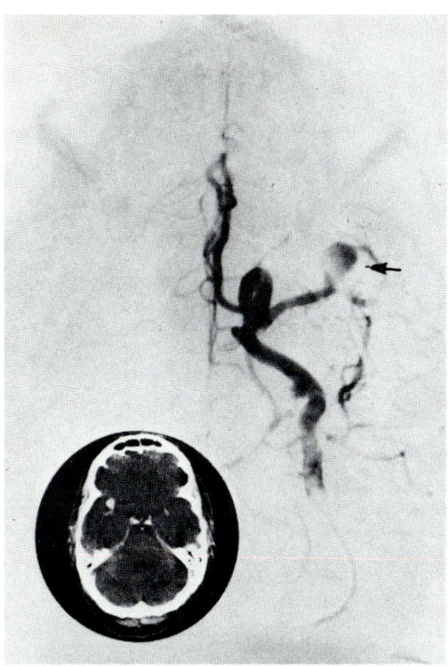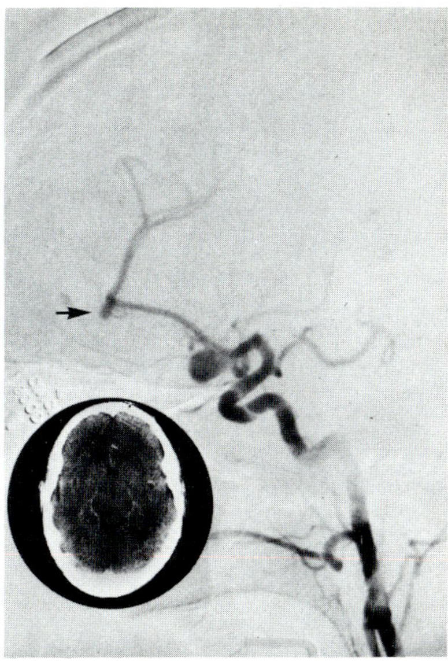

FIG. 6. High resolution CT scan demonstrating **(left)** an unruptured 12 mm middle cerebral artery aneurysm, and **(right)** (higher section) a 6 mm pericallosal aneurysm which was the site of subarachnoid hemorrhage.

(e) Hypertension: There is no unanimity of opinion concerning hypertension's role in the development of intracranial aneurysms, although there is little doubt that hypertension is associated with an aggravation of most degenerative vascular lesions (55). Recurrent hemorrhage from aneurysms is most closely related to uncontrolled hypertension (24). Hypertension must be a critical factor in patients with any of the other risk factors which augment aneurysmal formation (55).

(f) Familial aneurysms: The familial relationship is too infrequent to substantiate the existence of a familial disorder of the vascular wall (7). *Formes frustes* of connective tissue disorders, history of vascular accidents, and sites of occurrence of aneurysms, may be correlated in relatives.

SCREENING OF HIGH-RISK PATIENTS

On the basis of the documented warning signs and the conditions associated with increased incidence of intracranial aneurysms, we recommend the following guidelines for screening of high-risk individuals:

1. Computer scan with contrast enhancement with thin cuts if any of the conditions that have been associated with aneurysm are present in persons with reasonable health and life expectancy.

2. Angiography should be performed if the CT scan demonstrates an aneurysm larger than 5 mm in diameter.

3. If there is historical or clinical evidence of previous SAH recently or remotely.

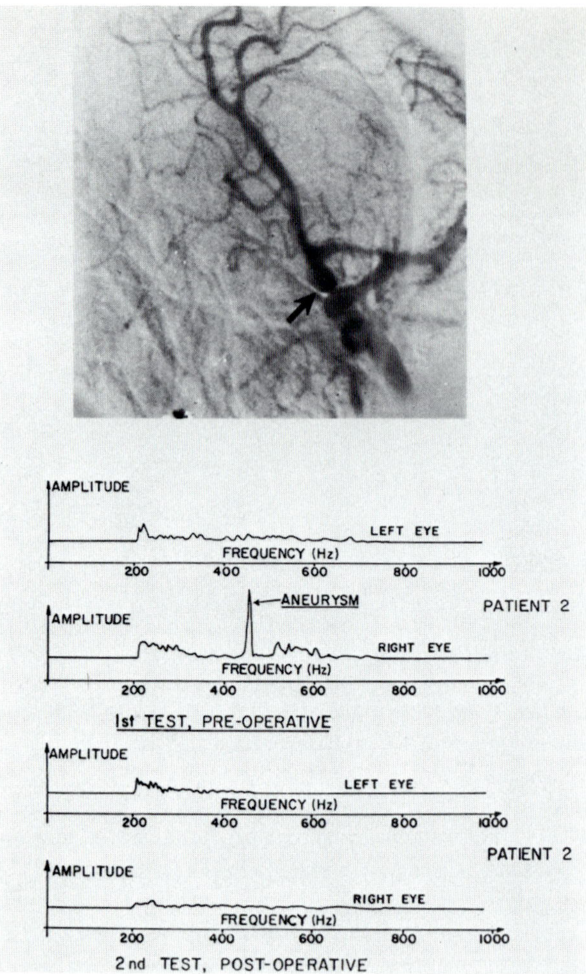

FIG. 7. Acoustical recording of internal carotid aneurysm. **Top:** In the pre-operative test, marked turbulence (right eye) is caused by internal carotid aneurysm. **Bottom:** The disturbance is completely absent in the post-operative test, after the aneurysm has been clipped. (From Olinger and Wasserman, ref. 36, with permission.)

4. If there has been a previous or ruptured aneurysm inadequately treated and if the total cerebral circulation has not been visualized by angiography. Multiple aneurysms occur in 20% of cases (46), (Fig. 6A,6B).

If the electronic stethoscope developed by Olinger (33) proves to be economically practical, it may provide a simple and effective method of investigating high-risk patients. This computer analysis system is capable of detecting minute variables in turbulence created by aneurysms of the internal carotid artery in or near the skull

TABLE 5. *Recommendations for screening patients for intracranial aneurysms*

1. History suggestive of prior SAH or warning symptoms
2. Documented fibromuscular dysplasia
3. Polycystic renal artery disease
4. Ehler-Danlos syndrome, pseudoxanthoma elasticum, Marfan's syndrome, aortic defects
5. Hypertension-headache?
6. Family history?

TABLE 6. *Screening procedure for intracranial aneurysm*

1. Careful history
2. Physical examination
3. Electronic stethoscope
4. CAT scan—contrast
5. Venous subtraction angiography
6. Cerebral angiography

TABLE 7. *Factors in determining advisability of operation for unruptured aneurysms*

1. Age and physiological condition of the patient
2. Size and location of the aneurysm
3. Signs or symptoms of enlargement or impending rupture
4. Experience of the treatment team
5. Opinion of the patient

base. The device is thus capable of screening the areas which are not subject to survey by the CT scan (Fig. 7).

A new technique, venous subtraction angiography, is capable of demonstrating large intracranial aneurysms (1 cm or greater), and improved technology may lead to replacement of arterial injection in some circumstances.

When the latent risks of a disease are as great as those documented by the natural history of SAH from intracranial aneurysm and if surgical treatment is the only acceptable form of curative treatment, it is appropriate to initiate a screening process for high-risk patients (Tables 5 and 6). Drake (13) has concluded that the intact aneurysm is not innocent. His follow-up demonstrated that 17% of untreated intact aneurysms ruptured. He reported no deaths and morbidity of 1.7% in the course of operation on 289 unruptured aneurysms in 246 patients (12). Mount (30) and Heiskanen (19) found that 10% of patients with unruptured aneurysms bled and 4% died within 5 years of initial diagnosis. Salazar (50) operated on 106 aneurysms in 78 patients with no deaths and 3% morbidity. Similar results have been reported from other centers (51).

The hope for the future lies in prevention (Table 7). In order to accomplish this, we must educate the public and the general physician about the importance of warning signs of impending SAH. This effort requires continued discussion of the problem at the public level, in medical schools, and in continuing education forums (61). Progressive reduction in the ravages of hypertension and occlusive cerebrovascular disease illustrates the benefits of this approach. The potential for preventing death and disability from cerebral aneurysm is considerable. Statistics indicate that approximately 30,000 persons suffer SAH annually in North America. The data indicate that at least 50% (15,000) die and another 25% are permanently disabled (13). Recognition of the aneurysm-prone patient can be achieved by selected screening tests. Skilled total management of mortality and morbidity is available throughout the country to reduce these figures to negligible levels. The challenge is obvious and the problem eminently manageable (34).

REFERENCES

1. Adams, H. P., Jergenson, D. O., Kassell, N. F., and Sahs, A. L. (1980): Pitfalls in the recognition of subarachnoid hemorrhage. *J. A. M. A.*, 244:794–796.
2. Allcock, J. M., and Canham, P. B. (1976): Angiographic study of the growth of intracranial aneurysms. *J. Neurosurg.*, 45:617–621.
3. Allcock, J. M. and Drake, C. G. (1965): Ruptured intracranial aneurysms. The role of arterial spasm. *J. Neurosurg.*, 21:21–29.
4. Antunes, J. L., and Carrell, S. W. (1976): Cerebral emboli from intracranial aneurysms. *Surg. Neurol.*, 6:7–10.
5. Bergin, J. J. (1966): The complication of therapy with epsilon-aminocaproic acid. *Med. Clin. North Am.*, 50:1669–1698.
6. Brown, R. A. P. (1951): Polycystic disease of the kidneys and intracranial aneurysms. The etiology and interrelationship of these conditions: Review of recent literature and report of seven cases in which both conditions coexisted. *Glasgow Med. So.*, 32:333–348.
7. Carroll, R. E., and Haddon, W. (1964): Birth characteristics of persons dying of intracranial aneurysms. *J. Chronic Dis.*, 17:705–711.
8. Crompton, M. R. (1964): Cerebral infarction following rupture of cerebral berry aneurysm. *Brain*, 87:263–280.
9. Dandy, W. E. (1944): *Intracranial Arterial Aneurysms*. Comstock, Ithaca, N. Y.
10. Davis, J. M., Davis, K. R., and Crowell, R. M. (1980): Subarachnoid hemorrhage secondary to ruptured intracranial aneurysm: Prognostic significance of cranial CT. *Am. J. Roentgenol.*, 134:711–715.
11. Dott, N. M. (1933): Cerebral arterioradiography. Surgical treatment. *Edin. Med. J.*, 40:219–240.
12. Drake, C. G. (1981): Progress in cerebral vascular disease: Management of cerebral aneurysm. *Stroke*, 12:273–283.
13. Drake, C. G., and Girvin, J. P. (1976): The surgical treatment of subarachnoid hemorrhage in multiple aneurysms. In: *Controversies in Neurosurgery*, edited by T. P. Morley, pp. 274–278. W. B. Saunders, Philadelphia.
14. Eisentrout, C., Tomsick, T. A., and Tew, J. M. (1980): Computed tomography findings as a prognostic factor in subarachnoid hemorrhage. *Stroke*, 11:124.
15. Fisher, M., Davidson, R. I., and Marcus, E. M. (1980): Transient focal cerebral ischemia as a presenting manifestation of unruptured cerebral aneurysm. *Ann. Neurol.*, 8:367–372.
16. Fisher, C. M., Kistler, J. P., and Davis, J. M. (1980): Relation of cerebral vasospasm to subarachnoid hemorrhage visualized by computerized tomographic scanning. *Neurosurgery*, 6:1–9.
17. Gillingham, F. J. (1958): The management of ruptured intracranial aneurysm. *Ann. R. Coll. Surg. Engl.*, 23:89–90.
18. Gillingham, F. J., (1967): The management of ruptured intracranial aneurysm. *Scott. Med. J.*, 12:377–381.
19. Heiskanen, O., and Martilla, I. (1970): Risk of rupture of a second aneurysm in patients with multiple aneurysms. *J. Neurosurg.*, 32:295–299.
20. Hoffman, W. F., Wilson, C. B., and Townsend, J. J. (1979): Recurrent transient ischemic attacks secondary to an embolizing saccular middle cerebral artery aneurysm. *J. Neurosurg.*, 51:103–106.

21. Hunt, W. E., and Koshik, E. J. (1974): Timing and perioperative care for intracranial aneurysm surgery. *Clin. Neurosurg.*, 21:79–89.
22. Hunt, W. E., and Miller, C. A. (1979): The results of early operation for aneurysm. *Clin. Neurosurg.*, 24:208–215.
23. Ito, U., and Inaba, Y. (1979): Cerebrospinal fluid cytology after subarachnoid hemorrhage. *J. Neurosurg.*, 57:352–354.
24. Jane, J. A. (1980): Natural history of subarachnoid hemorrhage: Reappraisal of need for surgery. In: *The Aneurysm Patient, Preoperative and Postoperative Care*, edited by L. N. Hopkins. Raven Press, New York.
25. King, R. B., and Saba, M. I. (1974): Forewarnings of major subarachnoid hemorrhage. *N. Y. State J. Med.*, 74:638–639.
26. Kraÿenbuhl, H. A., Yasargil, M. G., Flamm, E. S., and Tew, J. M. (1972): Microsurgical treatment of intracranial sacular aneurysms. *J. Neurosurg.*, 27:678–686.
27. Locksley, H. B. (1966): Natural history of subarachnoid hemorrhage, intracranial aneurysms and A-V malformations. *J. Neurosurg.*, 25:321–368.
28. McCormick, W. F. (1971): Natural history of intracranial aneurysms: Necropsy study. In: *Problems and Pathogenesis of Intracranial Aneurysms*, edited by S. Moosy, and R. Janeway, pp. 219–231. Grune and Stratton, New York.
29. McKissock, W., Paine, K. W. E., and Walsh, L. S. (1960): An analysis of treatment of ruptured intracranial aneurysms: Report of 772 consecutive cases. *J. Neurosurg.*, 17:762–776.
30. Mount, L. A., and Brisman, R. (1974): Treatment of multiple aneurysms—symptomatic and asymptomatic. *Clin. Neurosurg.*, 21:166–170.
31. Mullen, S., Hanlon, K., and Brown, F. (1978): Management of 136 consecutive supratentorial berry aneurysms. *J. Neurosurg.*, 49:794–804.
32. Nibbelink, D. W., Thorner, S. C., and Henderson, W. G. (1975): Intracranial aneurysms and subarachnoid hemorrhage. A cooperative study. *Stroke*, 6:622–629.
33. Nishimoto, A. (1979): Incidence of subarachnoid hemorrhage. Presented at the Japanese Neurological Society, Tokyo.
34. Ojemann, R. G. (1981): Management of the unruptured intracranial aneurysm. *N. Eng. J. Med.*, 304:725.
35. Okawara, S. H. (1973): Warning signs prior to rupture of an intracranial aneurysm. *J. Neurosurg.*, 38:575–580.
36. Olinger, C. P., and Wasserman, J. F. (1977): Electronic stethoscope for detection of cerebral aneurysm, vasospasm, and arterial disease. *Surg. Neurol.*, 8:298–312.
37. Pakarinen, S. (1967): Incidence, etiology of primary subarachnoid hemorrhage. *Acta. Neurol. Scand. (Suppl.)*, 43:1–128.
38. Palubinskas, A. J., Perloff, D., and Newton, T. H. (1966): Fibromuscular hyperplasia, an arterial dysplasia of increasing clinical importance. *Am. J. Roentgenol.*, 98:907–914.
39. Park, B. E. (1979): Spontaneous subarachnoid hemorrhage complicated by communicating hydrocephalus. *Surg. Neurol.*, 11:73–79.
40. Phillips, L. H., Whisnant, J. P., O'Fallon, W. P., and Sundt, T. M. (1980): The unchanging pattern of subarachnoid hemorrhage in a community. *Neurology*, 30:1034–1040.
41. Pool, J. L. (1959): Early treatment of ruptured intracranial aneurysms of the Circle of Willis with special clip technique. *Bull. N. Y. Acad. Med.*, 35:357–369.
42. Post, K. D., Flamm, E. S., Goodgold, A., and Ransohoff, J. (1977): Ruptured intracranial aneurysms: Case morbidity and mortality. *J. Neurosurg.*, 46:290–295.
43. Rhoton, A. L. (1978): Improving ourselves and our specialty. *Clin. Neurosurg.*, 26:13–19.
44. Roach, M. R. (1978): A model study of why some intracranial aneurysms thrombose but others rupture. *Stroke*, 9:583–587.
45. Rubinstein, M. K., and Cohen, N. H. (1964): Ehlers-Danlos syndrome associated with multiple intracranial aneurysms. *Neurology*, 14:125–129.
46. Sahs, A. L., Perret, G. E., Locksley, H. B., and Nishioka, H. (1969): Results of aneurysm treatment by intracranial surgery, carotid ligation, and bed rest in defined groups of patients. In: *Intracranial Aneurysms and Subarachoid Hemorrage*, pp. 245–275. Lippincott, Philadelphia.
47. Saito, I., and Sano, K. (1979a): Vasospasm following rupture of cerebral aneurysms. *Neurol. Med. Chir. (Tokyo)*, 19:103–107.
48. Saito, I., and Sano, K. (1979b): Symposium on timing of operation for ruptured aneurysms. Presented at the Japan Neurosurgical Society, Tokyo.

49. Sakaki, T., Kinugawa, K., Tanigake, T., Miyamoto, F., Kyor, K., and Utasumi, S. (1980): Embolism from intracranial aneurysms. *J. Neurosurg.*, 53:300–304.
50. Salazar, J. L. (1980): Surgical treatment of asymptomatic and unidentified intracranial aneurysms. *J. Neurosurg.*, 53:20–21.
51. Sampson, D. S., Hodash, R. M., and Clark, W. K. (1977): Surgical management of unruptured asymptomatic aneurysms. *J. Neurosurg.*, 46:731–734.
52. Sampson, D. S., Hodash, R. M., Reid, W. R., Beyer, C. W., and Clark, W. K. (1979): Risk of intracranial aneurysm surgery in the good grade patient: Early versus late operation. *Neurosurgery*, 5:422–426.
53. Shucart, W. A., Hussain, S. K., and Cooper, P. R. (1980): Epsilon-aminocaproic acid and recurrent subarachnoid hemorrhage. *J. Neurosurg.*, 53:28–31.
54. Slosberg, P. S. (1979): Zero percent mortality due to recurrent hemorrhage in follow-up of medically treated ruptured single intracranial aneurysms: A 23-year study. *Trans. Am. Neurol. Assoc.*, 104:180–183.
55. Stehbens, W. E. (1972): In: *Pathology of the Cerebral Blood Vessels*. Mosby, St. Louis.
56. Stewart, R. M., Sampson, D., Diehl, S., Hinton, R., and Ditmore, Q. M. (1980): Unruptured cerebral aneurysms presenting as recurrent transient neurologic deficits. *Neurology*, 30:47–57.
57. Sundt, T. M., Jr., and Whisnant, J. P. (1978): Subarachnoid hemorrhage from intracranial aneurysms. Surgical management and natural history of the disease. *N. Engl. J. Med.*, 299:116–122.
58. Suzuki, J., Yoshimoto, T., and Okuma, T. (1978): Early operations for ruptured intracranial aneurysms. *Neurol. Med. Chir. (Tokyo)*, 18:83–89.
59. Symonds, C. P. (1924): Spontaneous subarachnoid hemorrhage. *Q. J. Med.*, 18:93–107.
60. Tyler, H. R., and Clark, D. B. (1958): Neurological complications in patients with coarctation of aorta. *Neurology*, 8:712–718.
61. Wiebers, D. O., Whisnant, J. P., and O'Fallon, W. M. (1981): The natural history of unruptured intracranial aneurysms. *N. Engl. J. Med.*, 304:696–698.
62. Yasargil, M. G. (1969): In: *Microsurgery Applied to Neurosurgery*. George Thieme, Verlag, Stuttgart.
63. Yasargil, M. G., and Fox, J. L. (1975): The microsurgical approach to intracranial aneurysms. *Surg. Neurol.*, 3:7–14.
64. Zacks, D. J., Russell, D. B., and Miller, J. D. R. (1980): Fortuitously discovered intracranial aneurysms. *Arch. Neurol.*, 37:39–41.

Subject Index